Journey of Seven Steps

Jyoti Joshi

© Copyright 2021 Jyoti Joshi

No parts of this publication may be reproduced by any means without the express written permission of the author.

ISBN: 978-0-578-30363-5

To Madhukar, my Raja.

And to all caregivers out there.

Life isn't about waiting for the storm to pass. It's about learning how to dance in the rain. - Vivian Greene

Prologue

When Madhukar and I were getting married, we did a ritual called Saptapadi - seven times we walked together around the sacred fire, my hand in his, as we recited promises to each other. Thus begin our everlasting relationship said to continue into our next seven lives. I was too young and naive to imagine where those steps would take me.

Because of his kind nature and zest for life, Madhukar became my sun and moon. The rays of our happiness were immeasurable. Our glass was always full. And for 47 years, our four feet marched together as a team. But suddenly two feet stumbled, and his firm grip on my hands became frail.

My Sun and the moon were eclipsed. Madhukar became a victim of Alzheimer's disease[1].

My mother's childhood friend Malu Auntie's, favorite mantra was, 'Life is like an ocean's tides. Never get depressed experiencing low tides, because immediately the high tides will follow.' I used to listen to her discourses on Sri Ramakrishna Paramahamsa. It influenced me to Indian philosophy when I was in college. Later in life his teachings helped me tremendously. So did her pearls of wisdom buried deep in my heart.

'I love life' was always my Mantra. But after the doctor revealed his illness, black clouds of negativity surrounded me. All I saw was the tsunami of his suffering. Madhukar's mind was fuming with chaos;

---

[1] By 2025, the number of people age 65 and older with Alzheimer's disease is estimated to reach 7.1 million, a 140% increase from the more than 5 million who are currently affected. Every 7 second there is an Alzheimer's diagnosis. - Alzheimer's Association's calendar

the darkness of his confusion started covering my mind too. Like the mid-day sun, this fiery illness started scorching me, and I desperately looked for refuge.

Caring for Madhukar brought me humility. I became keenly aware that I was surrounded by gurus, and I was grateful for their wisdom. It became the most spiritual experience I ever had in my life, though of course I didn't realize it at the time.

As in a gusty rainstorm, an umbrella would fly away, in the turmoil of Alzheimer's Madhukar flew far away from me into an unknown world. My path became constantly uphill huge cliffs of his dementia. Until then we were always together on our beautiful voyage, but because of his illness, this journey was now mine alone.

My fatigued mind and body took shelter in mother nature's beauty. Slowly, it calmed me down like a cool breeze in the midst of desolation. My feet could feel the soft grass on my rocky path, and this would give me new strength to face all the challenges. The light at the end of the tunnel became visible.

Writing in my diary took on new importance as well. It was already a lifelong habit, but now it also became a hidden armor against the monstrous disease's onslaught. Without fail, I started writing in my journal every day. The diary became my *sathi,* companion, while the pen became my sword. As soon as I wrote about the day's difficult task, I was able to separate myself from that particular heartache. It was extremely beneficial for my mental stability. Yet all that time, I had a feeling somebody else was writing through me. I was just a *nimit matra,* a conduit. Writing gave me the capacity to observe myself with
Sakshi-bhavana, simply be a witness.

But still sometimes, Madhukar's unbearable suffering would crack my strength, and I would become 'Jyoti-wife-caregiver' again. So I decided to keep '*Jyoti-me-i-she*' purposely in all those roles in my writings.

When I tried to fathom Madhukar's suffering and put it into writing, it became like Pandora's box. The tears would wipe away my words.

It was too excruciating to even try to imagine what he must be going through. So I have written only about my own experiences. My life is ordinary, but what if I too lost my memory and forgot what I was dealing with? So I started writing my memoirs. I realized that there are so many caregivers like me who are taking care of loved ones through this unimaginable and incurable disease. They must have some of the same feelings. Maybe they could identify with my journey, and my experience might be a small lantern on their road ahead.

'Yadvācā'nabhyuditaṃ yena vāgabhyudyate ... yanmanasā na manute yenāhurmano matam tadeva brahma tvaṃ viddhi nedaṃ yadidamupāsate.'- Kena Upanishad: 1-4,5

'What speech cannot reveal, but what reveals speech, that alone is Brahman ... What mind does not comprehend, but what comprehends the mind, that alone is Brahman, and not that which people worship.'

I surrender to that Brahman and give this book to you, the reader.

Jyoti Joshi
January 12, 2021

Based on my original book written in Marathi

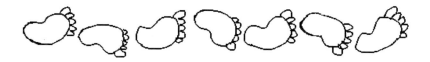

A Journey of Seven Steps

A journey of million footsteps…carrying so many precious memories. Which one to choose?

January 12, 1967

He holds her hand to walk seven steps together for *Saptpadi*. She feels the soft touch through his firm grip. It floods a gentle wave in her body. He repeats after the priest…

"Sakha saptapadi bhav – Let us remain true companions. Let us acquire knowledge, happiness and harmony by mutual love and trust… Now that you have taken seven steps with me, you are mine and I am yours for eternity. Please stay always with me, deeply rooted to give me support as a rock."

"Are you convinced now at last?" he comes closer and whispers in her ear. She could feel his breath, the color of her red sari mirrored on her face. His act was clearly visible to others. Wedding *Mandap*- full of guest, priest chanting mantras and the loud melody of *Shehnai*. She hopes no one heard him.

'How in the world have I married this proper stranger? Really? Who is he?'

Her mind clogs with all the qualms. Her hand unknowingly fidgets on *Mangalsutra*, her wedding necklace of black beads to keep the evils away symbolizing his enduring commitment to her. From now on she will have to wear it always.

After three brief meetings, today she became Mrs. Madhukar Joshi. Just like that!

***

June 24, 2012

He was restless since morning.

"Let's go out," she suggested, hoping he will feel better once he is out.

She drove him to Borderland State Park. She never liked calling it a park. Its far more that the park… lush flora and fauna… paths by the lake side. They have often walked there. She was sure that the scenic area would calm his mind.

His babbling continued all through the ride. But as soon as she parked the car in the parking lot suddenly, he became very uneasy and abruptly stopped talking.

She ignored his silence and held his hand firmly encouraging him to get out of the car, and said to him, "Let's walk down to our favorite place." She pointed at the pond. "Look our rock is waiting for us. Should we sit there first and just watch the birds?"

"Where are you taking me?" he demanded.

She was shocked; he did not recognize Borderland. She hauled him down the path toward the lake…Maybe when he sees the water lilies he will remember.

Wherever they went in the world, he would always remember every road and map as if it were carved in his mind. He had a photographic memory.

"I don't remember this road. I think we are lost," he murmured. He stared blankly as if he had never seen this park. This new change alarmed her.

She started showing him the familiar signs of surroundings, "oh look our rock and your beautiful red maple next to it." Still he was like a lost child with a timid look. The teacher in her took over, she convinced him that he was safe and took hold of his hand again and started walking. There was deep preserved forest behind their house. He would often say, let me take you into a magical world… and start walking there pulling her hand. Seeing her apprehension he would say don't worry, I have a magical wand *"Raja,* when you are holding my hand, I don't need any magical wand." She would lovingly answer him back.

"I am lost. I am lost. We are lost…"

"I love to get lost when your hand is in my hand."

"This is not the right way. Definitely we are on the wrong road!"

"When you are holding my hand, *I want to go on the road less traveled."*

"I'm fearful…I am really scared!"

"When your hand is in my hand, my fear dissolves! My hand is in your hands! Your hand is in my hand. That is our magic wand."

"I hate this road…look how many bumps and potholes are here."

"Raja, that's the real skill, we have to jump over all these hurdles. Did you see the beautiful water lilies? The honeybees have immersed themselves inside the lilies?"

"No I don't see any beauty… all I see is the horse's shit. I don't like walking here."

"The tall trees, their shade is keeping us cool. Listen, the cardinal is cooing to his mate…his sweet song. Isn't this romantic?"

"No no, I really can't hear that…we are completely lost Jyoti."

The forest ranger was trotting on his horse. She purposely asked him loudly, "Sir, is this the right path?"

"Yes Ma'am, you are on the correct path. This park is very safe," the Ranger assured them.

But that assurance did not help to calm him down. The same broken record again…

"Jyoti, I am scared… really afraid." Looked like he was about to cry.

She stopped in the middle of the road, stroked his back gently. Then held his hand again and turned around to go back home. He was still brooding, did not utter a single word on the way home.

She pushed on the remote to open the garage door impatiently. Ran inside and hurriedly started reading the Alzheimer's book that she had just brought from the library yesterday. Pages fluttered. So many rules for care givers…

- In this illness, whatever the patient expresses, those are his real experiences even though it is not reality. Don't try to convince him otherwise.
- Don't differ with him and support him with gentle assurance.
- Don't ridicule him or question him. Go with the flow.
- Distract him with positive statements and always encourage him.

Now she was very scared. She felt very guilty for making him walk on that road. She realized from now on she will have to constantly watch herself to not step over him and to communicate with tender loving words.

***

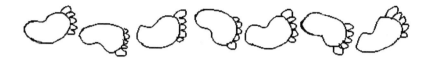

Through time, I've learned to accept what is. I've made a commitment to live for today. I'll do only what I can for the moment, and I'll continue to walk through the rainbow and add color wherever I can. - Marge Barnhart

September 12, 2013

The kettle on the stove started shrieking. Microwave's alarm was nagging. Milk is ready... Milk is ready. He likes warm milk for the tea. In the background, washer was loudly churning the clothes.

This is how her morning starts every day. His breakfast was almost ready. She needed to hurry up. Her heart ached! How she wished, in that very moment if only he could be his old self again.

She remembered the good old days... they had just settled into their very first home in America. The girls were still toddlers. They would be running around in the house. She would be busy cooking for dinner. The dishwasher would be on with a loud annoying clamor. The phone would ring at that exact moment...And at that noisy moment her darling husband would walk in the kitchen with a book in his hands,

"Jyoti, listen to this lovely poem."

"Raja, is this the time... for poetry? In the middle of this havoc? Who will cook dinner then?" she used to get annoyed.

Ignoring all her complaints he would start reciting the poem to her. After listening to him, all her anger would melt away into admiration for him. She would thank the goddess for tying the silk thread, a love of poetry, around them. When they were newlywed, they used to go together by a local train every day he to his office and she to her art school. Train would be packed with the morning rush hour. They would be standing in the door so close to each other that she could feel his breath on her. Loud clatter of the tracks and all the crowd around them would not stop him, whispering a love poem into her ears… Even though she adored it she would feel so conscious of the surrounded crowd, who could easily hear him.

'What else would I need when you are reading me poetry?" she would murmur in his ears…

She drew the curtain to let the sun in. Flapping of the curtain, reality hit her. The outside sunshine was not going to brighten her mind. She wished that she could catch those days again in that dream catcher in the window.

"Why can't I be a time traveler, like Asimov's science fiction?" Another passion from their many common interests. Her heart ached.

She looked at the clock, she could not afford to be late again today for his day care center. Then her whole day would chug along like a goods train unable to catch up the speed. But now she knew it was going to be the same story as yesterday. She needed to get his lunch box ready, write a note to his nurse at the adult day care center about his sugar level, and get ready for her own swimming …all the mundane chores as usual. She felt helpless.

She started feeding him, oatmeal, soaked almond, blueberries with cinnamon and chia. After his breakfast she coxed him toward the TV room. She helped him to sit securely on the couch. Lately he was losing his balance. Sometimes he would miss the seat and fall down. As he sat, he started rubbing his hands constantly. She knew behind that another new habit there was a mute agitation of his mind. She also became restless.

She always lived in a moment enjoying all the beauty around her. But ever since his illness started, she was struggling to surrender into present moment. She put the *Atmshatakam -Bhajan* on CD. *Shankaracharya's* great discovery of *Brahman*.

"*Chitdanandruph Shivoham* ... I am the constant bliss!"

She started finishing her chores in the kitchen. But suddenly she stopped working. Dropped everything... and went to him. She held his hand gently and sat next to him.

"The chores will never be finished," she grumbled and started listening to the deep meaning of the *Shankara's* hymns.

"*Na Mantro Na Tirtha*... It's not in mantra not in tirtha-the holy water of Ganga. Neither in Veda scriptures, nor in penance."

"You will not find God in any of the rituals, not in duty, not in service, not in practice, not in chanting... he is nowhere but only within you. I am only that ultimate pure bliss."

This was her favorite hymns-ultimate truth! She had been listening all her life. She wondered, how did Shankara understand this at such a tender age of 10? Saint Kabir also says the same thing.

'When would you achieve it?' her mind complained.

She kept coming back to the same stubborn wish... why can't her husband become his old self again... ever smiling, enthusiastic, and full of life. Her eyes welled. Why can't I accept this new him?

She was entangled like a fly in the fragile fibers of his love...a fish out of water.... when will this *Maya* vanish? When would this greedy thirst quench?

She thought he was feeling safe holding her hand but then he let it go to the very next moment. Did the same over and over again. It was like a cat and mouse game,

The doctor kept telling her, he does not understand, his brain can't feel or express…but she was confident that he knew. She would be always there for him, holding his hand forever…her strong conviction.

'*I am the constant bliss.*'

The enchanting hymn empowered her. Like a magic, her mind blew the trumpet at that very moment.

'God? Where else he could be? He is candidly embedded right next to me in Madhukar's body… I did not see him at all before. Let all the doctrine be left aside! He is my only God now. There is nothing else in my world! No other agenda! I will never let go of his hand!'

She made a firm decision with herself. The grip of her hand on him became tight… She found a new way to communicate with him…only from her gentle soft touch.

***

November 23, 1966

"Jyoti, you must get married before I retire," everyday Dada's new Mantra will hammer her ears. "Why such a hurry Dada?" She would beg her father. She did not even finish unwrapping all the gifts he gave her yesterday on her 20th birthday. Nowadays, there was just only one discussion in the household… Jyoti's wedding. Her mother-*Aai* was also constantly on the hunt for an eligible bachelor for Jyoti.

Jyoti was the least interested in getting married. She was dreaming about going to Paris or Italy for her Master's in arts after she finished this last year of art school. Sunita, her girlfriend from college, was also collaborating in this secret plan. But now she was feeling helpless against her father's decision.

Dada's younger brother Dattu died suddenly few months ago, the whole family was shaken by this blow. Everybody lovingly called him "*Baba*" which means father. He was indeed a second father to her.

Now Dada was responsible for Dattu's family – Sumati, his young widow whom all the young ones called *Akka* (elder sister), and her three children. Theirs was a typical joint family. There was no separation between siblings and cousins.

If there is a death in the family, weddings or other sacred ceremonies have to take place within the year. Otherwise one has to wait three years. That's why Dada was determined to get Jyoti married before the year was over.

Shanta Aunty came to visit one afternoon. She was Jyoti's favorite aunt. Shanta Aunty's attire was a very simple, just like her innocent loving nature. She would always bring Jyoti's favorite *Dalimbya*, spicy legumes. Today was no exception. "Kamal," she called as soon as she entered the house. That was Aai's maiden name. Jyoti loved that name. Lotus flower. But nobody would call her mother by that name; it was twisted into Kamutai. Her Aai was the oldest of her 5 siblings. So Tai was added to Kamu out of respect. Shanta and Kamal were together since grade school; their friendship was thicker than blood. Shanta Aunty started telling her Aai before she even took her chappals from her feet. "Hey Kamal, I know a very good eligible bachelor. We were interested for our daughter Malati. But found out only this morning that their horoscopes don't match. That's why I came to you urgently. He is foreign-returned from America. He just bought a flat in *Dombivali*. Before that they used to live in *Palan Sushapal*. Why don't you try him for Jyoti?" Those words annoyed Jyoti. She could not believe Shanta Aunty's logic. Getting married is not like buying sandals or a blouse from the store. If that sandal does not fit Malati, maybe it will fit Jyoti??

Two days after that, her Aai was on a local train traveling the long distance to Dombivali to check out the bachelor. A conflict started boiling in her mind. The bachelor's name was Madhukar Joshi. She did not want to marry somebody with the last name *Joshi*. The name was so common! And his first name was Madhukar! She hated that name because there were two Madhukar she already knew who lived down the street. They had never made any impression on her. Her Aai's uncle lived in Dombivali and she did not enjoy her visits there. Jyoti shuddered. She felt nauseous by just the thought of the stench of open sewage in Dombivali. With all these negative factors, why were Aai and Dada even considering this boy? She was very angry. But she knew her opinion does not count, being the youngest in the family. "Maybe my horoscope also won't match. That will be a Godsend," Jyoti muttered. She was happy to hear what her Aai told Dada about her saga to visit the Joshi family. Her Aai realized that she knew Madhukar's mother. They both belonged to the same *Samiti,* women's organization. After explaining the reason why she came to visit, his mother told her that they have already found a future bride for Madhukar and both parties were meeting on the very same afternoon, that day. Dada and Aai were very disappointed but Jyoti was relieved with delight.

The next day was a typical Sunday afternoon. Jyoti was sweeping the floor. Her sari pulled to her knees. Humidity in the air was unbearable. Her face was drenched. Her hair was a mess. The doorbell rang. Their house was always busy with company. She opened door without even thinking of her appearance. A couple was standing at the threshold. The lady introduced herself, "I am Mrs. Apte, Madhukar Joshi's Aunt." Jyoti let them in and pointed at the sofa in the living room. Dada entered the room. Mrs. Apte continued with the purpose of her visit. "Yesterday the marriage meeting at Joshi's house never took place. A telegram came from the girl's father... the girl did not have the courage to tell her parents that she did not want to marry anybody else because she already had a boyfriend. So Madhukar is willing to meet your daughter. You can give me her horoscope to see if there is a match." Before Jyoti could comprehend, Dada rushed to his desk and handed Jyoti's horoscope to Mrs. Apte.

Within the next few days, everything happened like a fast-forward tape. Her horoscope was a perfect match to Madhukar. Dada returned home very impressed after he met Madhukar in his office at the *Jamnalal Bajaj,* a prestigious Institute. He was carrying Madhukar's biodata in his hand. He proudly told the family that Madhukar came first for his *M.Sc.* class and won a gold medal in Mumbai University. He went for further studies to the US at Case Western University in Cleveland. After earning his doctorate degree in the statistics he returned home. Now he was teaching 'operation research' at business management at Bajaj Institute. 'Operation Research'? Everybody was puzzled in the house. Nobody knew what it meant. Jyoti was suddenly felt a big relief… her art school was not compatible to his brilliant career. So surely, he will not be interested in meeting her.

Dada kept talking about Madhukar's future plans. He was returning right back to America after the marriage. A particular important job was waiting for him. Madhukar warned Dada that he might not want his only daughter to go far away to a foreign country. Dada assured him, that will not be the case since his niece Usha has already gone to America, so he was used to the idea.

"By the way, Jyoti he was very much impressed by your fine arts choice." Dada's words lingered in her mind.

Dada asked Jyoti how she felt about Madhukar being 8 years older than her. "I will decide after I meet him personally," she replied with a sigh.

Once in a while she would hear or read in the paper that some chap got married and went abroad for further studies. Mostly abroad was USA. It was considered a high honor. But she had never heard about anybody going there for a job. Everybody in the house was excited that she would get a chance to go to America. Jyoti was a little curious about America after reading Ushatai's letters. Still, her ambition was strong only to go to Italy or Paris, rather than America.

Dada started inquiring into the Joshi family's background and found out that their financial status was not as good as he would have wanted for his daughter. Madhukar's father was a patriot and had dedicated his life to the freedom movement as a young man. As a result, he had ignored his own personal life and did not finish his education. So, he became a tailor. Ironically, British Sahibs would come to him for custom-made tailored suits.

"Do you really want Jyoti to live like that?" One of the uncles questioned Dada about this vast difference in the Joshi lifestyle.
Dada asked Jyoti how she felt about this. She gave her answer, "Dada, if this young man has earned his Ph.D. in America and with a job in hand, I don't think I will starve. I am not marrying his family's estate." "*Pori* (my little girl), you are so wise!" Dada's voice trembled

as he patted her back in approval. Somehow his compliment did not do the usual trick. She knew there was no other way out than to meet this so-called good catch.

Usually the boy's family would visit and would observe the girl as she served tea to the boy's family. She never liked this idea of displaying herself. 'I would like to meet him somewhere outside the home," she told Dada firmly. The next day Dada called Madhukar, who agreed immediately to meet her in the newly opened *Resham Bhavan* tea shop in Church gate at the other end of Bombay.

When Sumati, her best friend from college, heard the news she insisted that Jyoti wear her beautiful peacock blue chiffon sari for the occasion. Finally, the day arrived but she was still feeling ambivalent about this meeting. Jyoti went to Sumati's hostel directly from college. "Now remember, Dada will invite you in, but you have to refuse. I want to meet him alone," Jyoti warned Sumati as they were riding in a taxi.

As she entered Resham Bhavan, there was a different scenario. Her two elder brothers and their wives were standing near Dada. So meeting Madhukar alone was not going to happen! On top of that Dada insisted that Sumati should join them also. She was frustrated but obediently went inside hoping it is just a formality and nothing would come of it. There were two gentlemen sitting at the corner table. She recognized one of them. She had seen Madhukar's photo that Dada had brought home. Something strange happened; she realized that he didn't fit the mold of a 'Madhukar' but was in fact quite smart looking and handsome. He made a strong impression on her with his curly dark hair and sharp nose, and she liked his black-rimmed glasses in the latest style.

'A stranger has come to the door, yet it feels like I knew him in all of my lives'. A popular song started ringing in her ears…She could not understand what was happening. She was swept away; Madhukar in his blue suit took over her existence. Her eyelashes fluttered like a bird trying to escape. Her heart was beating so fast and loud, she was afraid he would hear it.

"Have we met before?" She was snapped out of the sweet enchanted magical moment. His voice was so soft. "No, I don't think so!" she answered hesitantly. Was he feeling the same way? "Are you sure?" he repeated, almost whispering. Now coming to her senses she firmly told him that no, she did not meet him before! Jyoti was amused by his low voice. Was he checking her hearing? She thought he was going to take out a needle and thread from his pocket to test her eyesight now! She had heard such funny stories from her *Vatsala Aaji*. Aaji was only 11 when she got married, which was a typical in the early 20th century.

He did not ask her any questions directly after that. The next hour went by quickly, a boring formal conversation among all of them. He left without saying goodbye or any further commitment to meet again. She was restless with uncertainty. She wanted so much to meet him alone. "He must give me a positive response. I want him to be my companion for the rest of my life," she confessed to Sumati helplessly.

***

"Jyoti wear a nice sari and get ready. We are going to my uncle. He has brought another proposal," Dada told her the following week. His uncle was very fond of Jyoti. This so-called eligible suitor came from a rich family. His father owned an airplane-part manufacturing plant. She was shocked by Dada's words. "Dada, please, I don't want to go see another boy. Let Madhukar at least give his answer," she begged Dada. She was glad to have Aai's support in this matter. But Dada had already committed. He would not go back on his promise made to his uncle. "*Pori*, this way you will have a choice. Be practical," Dada tried to convince her against her wishes. Dada and his practicality as usual left no room for choice for her. Her eyes teary, she bit her lip, put on her sandals angrily and started running down the stairs ahead of Dada without responding.

When they reached her uncle's place, there was no boy, only his mother and sister. They would approve her first and then the boy would come. He was flying home soon from his business commitment. She was annoyed to see how one woman could treat another woman as an object to be exhibited like this.

She was tortured by Madhukar's lack of immediate reply. How can he, the foreign-returned boy, be so mannerless? Finally, after a long week of agony she was relieved when Madhukar Joshi's affirmative answer came. With that, *not to get married before her finals, going to Venice for further studies,* all those dreams evaporated in the air. Meanwhile the other bachelor without even seeing her also sent his approval. Dada asked her, "Now what should we do?" "Tell the other boy to go fly away on the wings of the plane," she instantly chirped with joy.

Immediately on the following Sunday, Christmas eve, the *Baithak* was held to go over the marriage agreement between the two families. Jyoti was quite confident that Madhukar being highly educated and foreign returned there won't be much hassle about a dowry. His parents had not seen her yet, so the meeting was set in his new flat in Dombivali. Their apartment was in a brand-new building. Rice paddies behind the building, and a meadow in front, where some schoolboys were playing cricket and Madhukar was pitching the ball. The lush green color from rice paddies sprouted shoots in her mind of her future life with him. Gentle joy breezed her into a path of their happy life together. Madhukar rushed to enter the building before them as soon as he saw her family. She liked his stylish beige shirt with a checkered design.

The apartment was very spacious compared to Mumbai standards. Madhukar's mother and another gentleman greeted them in the leaving room. His father was in his bedroom. She bowed and touched his feet.

She was hoping to have a private chat with Madhukar in the other room to ask why he chose her. But she was disappointed when she saw Madhukar joined them for the meeting in the leaving room. It bothered her that he did not even say *'hello'* to her. Her Aai and she both left the house quickly to visit Aai's uncle nearby. Dada and Aai's uncle returned within an hour. On their return journey to Dadar, Dada started telling all the details of the *Baithak-meeting* to Aai. Madhukar was returning to America for his new job as soon as possible, so the *Muhurta* was chosen right away. She will be getting married within two weeks. Madhukar respectfully agreed to Aai's request that Jyoti should accompany him to the US and not go later on like other brides did in those days. Dada could not stop talking about the meeting. He beamed, 'the Joshi's did not demand a dowry', which made Jyoti happy, but the next sentence shocked her. "They asked us to take care of all the expenses of the wedding and requested that the bride would be adorned with (gold)ornaments." "Dada, what is this? Some kind of business contract? Nonsense? I do not agree to their demand," Jyoti raised her voice forgetting about the other train passengers. "*Pori* don't pay attention to these things. I am going to take care of it. All you should be concerned about is that you like the groom!" For the next few days Jyoti's mind was like a cloudy sky, unable to see the sun. She was hoping that she could convince Madhukar to change the terms if she could meet him personally.

Jyoti was attending the wedding of one of her childhood friends in Pune. Madhukar's uncle-*Kaka* and his wife *Kaku*, who were second parents to him, lived nearby and they wanted to meet Jyoti. Jyoti found out that they were traveling by train to Dombivali. She begged Achut Mama (maternal uncle), 'Please, can you book my ticket on the same train so I will have some company'? Achut Mama agreed to her request right away. They had a special bond between them ever since Achut Mama lived with them in Dadar when Jyoti was just a baby. She was pleased with her smart plan, hoping to steal some time on the train with Madhukar alone.

But that did not work out as Jyoti desired. Madhukar's Kaku was very orthodox and would not allow them to be unchaperoned. All they could do was to stand next to each other at the door of the compartment and admire the beautiful hills and valleys at Khandala Ghat. The train stopped at Dombivali station. The first-class compartment was far past the platform. His Kaka had suffered a stroke few years back, so he was unable to walk well. Madhukar was upset at the train authority for the lack of stairs and accommodations for the elderly and disabled. He did his best to help Kaka get down. Jyoti was touched by Madhukar's extreme care and tender help. She was hoping he would come back to her after assisting his uncle, but he was so absorbed in the process that he left without saying a word or even turning his head towards her. She wondered if he forgot, or was shy, or just did not care? *Who is this guy? I really don't know him that well. Am I making a mistake by committing my life to him in marriage?* There were lots of boys after her in college, but she did not care for any of them. She wanted to have a *love marriage*. At the very least she wanted to know Madhukar a little more closely and have a little friendship between them. Her two older brothers had gone out with their fiancés a few times before they got married. She wanted the same opportunity. She became very restless.

Next day she pleaded with Dada to let her go to a famous play with Madhukar. Dada hesitantly agreed on one condition, that her brother Aba and his wife would join them as chaperones. To her satisfaction Madhukar agreed right away. She had attended many concerts, movies, plays with her college friends, which included lots of boys, but this was different. She became impatient with glee. She could not decide what sari to wear, what jewelry would be fit for this occasion, that evening was going to add beautiful colors to her life. She braided jasmine *gajara* in her long silky black braid. Its fragrance burst in the air. Her peach color *chanderi* sari competed with the twilight.

Abhisarika excitedly lingered at the entrance of the theater. Her sister-in-law was teasing her. Madhukar had been out of the country for the last five years, so he didn't know where the newly built theater was. Aba was going to pick him up from his office. They were supposed to meet her at the door. Her eyes searched for Madhukar. Then she saw Aba walking hurriedly towards them, alone. Disappointment spread over her heart like a black cloud. Aba had gone to pick up Madhukar from his college as planned. Traffic was bad and he was a few minutes late. When he entered Madhukar's office, the room was empty. Aba waited for a while in vain, then he asked the custodian if he had seen Madhukar. The custodian looked around and then told him, his jacket is not on the chair, so he must have left already. Reluctantly Aba left, hoping Madhukar was on his way separately to the theater. All three went inside to their reserved seats. She was still hoping Madhukar would soon be sitting in the vacant seat next to her. The final bell rang indicating the opening of the curtain. Still no sign of Madhukar. She was glad nobody saw her face. Jasmine petals started dripping from her eyes. The love story of the drama was piercing to her already wounded heart.

***

Two days went by as she waited impatiently for his phone call. Why did he not bother to give any explanation to her? *'I really liked Madhukar from the moment I met him, but maybe he does not feel the same about me!'* the thought kept pricking her. *'How can he not want to know me more, the one who is going to spend an entire life with him? This is not the sign of an educated and sophisticated mind! The whole idea of marriage must have been against his wishes, just to please his parents.'* Her sleep was destroyed by this notion for a week.

She made up her mind resolutely that she would not hold the *varmala*[2] in her hands until she confronted him privately. "Dada, I want to talk to Madhukar in person, otherwise I won't marry him." "What's the matter with you, Jyoti? The invitations are already mailed, the wedding hall is booked, all the preparations are underway, why are you saying this now? What is the purpose of this meeting? What possible excuse can I give him?" Dada was stunned by her petition. "Why can't you just tell him the truth that I want to meet him again?" she demanded. Nobody took her side in the house. She felt so alone. "Listen, I have observed his manners, the boy is exceptional. Nothing wrong with him. Trust me, *Pori*," Dada tried to convince her in vain. In the end he gave up and went along with her decision. Next day he took her to Madhukar's office.

"You don't have to come upstairs. I want to see him alone," she meekly told Dada. "No, no, it doesn't look right!" he pushed the lift button for the floor quickly not giving her a choice.

***

The lift was going upward while her spirit was going down. *What if my doubt is correct and he really does not want to marry me?* There were some foreign-returned eligible bachelors nowadays with this trend. They are already married to white girls, but they do the marriage farce to stop the parent's nagging. She remembered her friend telling her of a similar episode recently. The lift door opened right in front of Madhukar's office, but her feet weakly lingered hesitantly. Dada entered his office announcing, "I needed the

---

[2] Varmala is a ceremony where the bride and groom exchange flower garlands symbolizing that they've accepted each other as life partners.

measurements of your ring finger." She was shocked to hear Dada's words. How could he add one more item to the already exorbitant wedding bill? She was bewildered by Madhukar's face-a grid full of questions upon seeing her. Not even a simple hello? She signaled Dada to leave the room. Dada took the measurement and reluctantly submitted to her gesture. Madhukar's friend, the same guy who had accompanied him to *Resham Bhavan*, was sitting in the room. She firmly looked at Madhukar, her voice stronger than her knees,

"I want to speak to you alone!" Madhukar was puzzled by her declaration. He motioned silently to his friend to leave the room.

"Are you marrying me against your wishes?" her words soared like a sharp arrow at him, yet she felt like a wounded prey herself. Madhukar stayed extremely quiet. Confused looks of indecision dipped across his face and destroyed her courage. She did not have the strength to hear his answer. The silence in the room was choking her.

"Why on earth do you have this strange notion?" at last he spoke.

"Well, you did not show up that evening at the play, nor did you bother to call the next day with at least an explanation. On the train your conversation was mundane. You never asked me to go out with you alone. Considering all this, I figured you are marrying me to please your parents," she burst out with all her enquiries in one breath.

"No, no, not at all. Nothing like that," he urged sincerely. On the evening of the play, I was waiting for your brother to pick me up. I waited for a long time, but he did not show. I assumed the plans had fizzled out. I would have taken a taxi but did not know the name of the theater. Believe me, I am not marrying you against my wishes. On the contrary…" He paused a moment. "There is no adult other than me in our house able to take care of all the preparations and get ready for wedding guest. And soon after the wedding, we will leave for America, so I have lot to take care of in that planning too. Really, I am all boggled with all this. No time for myself." His face crinkled with a smile. She was relieved to hear his explanation, stumbling at his pause with the words 'on the contrary'. She was hoping that he would take her out to a nearby cafe. She had kept the afternoon free. But he only walked with her to the VT station, explaining that he needed to buy a sack of rice for the coming guests.

'Shamma jalati hai to parwana chala ata hai- if the candle keeps flickering then moth would hover over it ... Jyoti means a tiny flame of light and Madhukar means honeybee.

'I wanted to choose a partner after falling in love with each other. That did not happen so now I will make Professor Madhukar Joshi fall in love with me after marriage!', she crooned to the loud beat of the iron wheels as the train left the station. The next week went by quickly in the jubilant celebration of her bridal showers, shopping, and mischievous teasing of her friends.

***

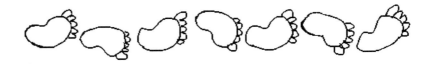

January 12, 1967

They got married on the perfect *muhurta* of the waxing crescent moon while *Shehnai* filled the *mandap* with joyous melodies. It was a festive ambience, everybody admiring how lovely the newlyweds looked. Eagerly waiting for the groom to feed his bride a mouthful of sweet *jilebi*. Madhukar surprised her with a gift in the middle of the ceremony. "That day when you entered my office, I was so impressed and delighted by your courage. For your valor, I am giving you these ruby *Tode,* bangles. Now please don't doubt me and always have faith that I have chosen you full-heartedly." She blushed at his honest confession and nodded speechlessly. She fed him *burfi*; thus began their sweet life together.

But the doubts still hover over her. *He is still a stranger to me. I don't know him. How will I find out who is truly hiding behind his biodata?* Her mind pondered, demanding, *'do you even know what exactly is identity? Is it likes and dislike? Is it his style? Is it the way he walks or talks?'*

***

'Babul mora naihar chhuto hi jaye'[3], - *Papa the shawl that you gave me is not ready to slip from my fingers-* started humming in her mind...

---

[3] The song was written by Nawab Wajid Ali Shah, the 19th-century Nawab of Awadh. A bride's farewell from her father- babul's home. It became very famous in concerts and Hindi movies.

With teary eyes, she bid farewell to Aai Dada. Today she would be leaving them behind to start her new life with her new unknown family. Overnight she would have to accept their new customs and be a dutiful daughter-in-law, wife, sister-in-law … so many roles to fit into. The walls of her new home felt so cold and strange.

Next day all the guests left. The house was very quiet. She kept busy unpacking her stuff. In the evening Madhukar suggested a walk to the border of the village. She was pleased to join him full heartedly, their very first walk together. The road curved alongside the railroad tracks. Madhukar pointed to a rock to sit on. "From childhood I have always been fascinated by the trains," he told her. For the next half, an hour all he talked about was trains: which train went where, which one would be coming next. He knew the timetable in detail. She was not interested in his commentary. She wanted to talk about their future. She wanted to know all about him. This was her first chance to get to know his true self. Again the same thought scolded her, *'Do you even know yourself? Have some patience.'* A train shrieked by, deafening her ears. "Did you bring me here just to talk about trains?" All he did was smile at her awkwardly. Soon they headed home.

After dinner, her in-laws retired early; fatigue from the wedding made them very tired. She started to look for something to read. Madhukar interrupted her, "Let me show you my slides from Europe." He had already set the slide projector up in the leaving room. He began to tell her about his trip. In the middle of the slideshow, she was overcome by giggles. He was puzzled by her laughter. All his photos were about pebbles, stones and rocks and nature! What was so funny about it?

On her mind's screen, projected an old incident: She started talking "One day I was arranging *Aboli*-Crossandra flowers in a copper dish. I needed something to support them, so I hurriedly went downstairs and grabbed a handful of small pebbles. Dada was standing nearby and tongue-in-cheek he said, "*Rikama nhavi ani kudyala tumadya lawi*" – the idle barber has nothing else to do so he keeps doing useless activities. Dada continued to mutter, "How in the world am I going to find you a husband as crazy as you who loves stones and rocks?"

She stared at Madhukar adoringly and murmured to herself, *'Today with Dada's help I have found that crazy man.'*

It was getting late. The evening melted into a starry night. She went to the bedroom and he hurriedly followed her; they were finally alone. He stood so close to her that she could hear his heartbeats. She didn't know what to do. There was a newspaper on the bedside table and she quickly snatched it up and pretended to read.

He took it away from her hand and held her chin toward him smiling at her playfully. "This is not the time to read the newspaper." His gaze locked onto hers. She blushed and the words slipped rescuing thousands of butterflies from her heart, "We really don't know each other, let's just talk tonight?"

He was amused by her plea. Not a moment passed by before he responded with a gentle but strong pledge, "Jyoti, we will be together for a lifetime, we have plenty of time. So don't worry. I will never force you ever to do anything. When I first saw you, in your college, your big amber eyes …you immediately captured my heart. I knew, my life would be entwined in the rainbow colors of you and your art. So don't worry, I have plenty of time. Let's talk heart-to-heart for eternity."

'So he can actually communicate!' she thought to herself. Moonbeams burst through her veins. All her doubts melted away by his sweet assurance, his promise like a sun shone through the dark clouds of her mind. She was dancing on a wave of ecstasy. She quickly realized, this was the side of him she had wanted to be introduced to, not his degree or reputation. The beautiful hues of his personality seeped all the way into her heart's palate.
"Why didn't you ask me out then, I would have skipped my classes and joined you! From now on I am going to call you *Raja*," she announced with glee.

"Pori, gone are the days of *Raja*-kings who always supported artists," Dada had warned when he heard of her headstrong decision to go to art school instead of medical school, against his wishes. In five years of college, there were lots of young budding artists wooing her.

But she was not interested in marring an artist. All she wanted was one true *rasik* who would relish her art.

Captivated in each other's embrace, their heart-to-heart talk, they did not know when Venus set, and dawn started.

***

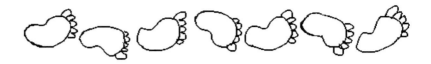

November 3, 1967

The dawn rose to a new horizon full of dreams. We were about to leave for the airport. Our *saptapadi* was multiplying from 7 to 10,000 steps with our journey to America, the Land of Gold. I had lived such a sheltered life as Aai Dada's youngest child, I had hardly ventured past Pune. Now the first time I was flying so far across the seven seas, leaving my parent's shelter. We were supposed to leave within a week after our wedding but ended up waiting a long nine months to get our green cards. Madhukar did not want to leave India without them. My soulmate at my side, I was not worried at all of the hardship awaiting us in the foreign land but instead was daydreaming about the glorious new life awaiting us in America. My foot lingered a bit yesterday as I left our new apartment in Dombivali. How quickly I got attached to a place of my very own. I had thrown my heart into decorating that apartment.

Aai did all the traditional rituals to send her daughter on such a long journey. With a solemn face, she put a spoonful of homemade *dahi* on my palms for me to lick, so that the taste of home would linger with me and I would not forget to return for a visit. Suddenly she held me tight to her bosom, and I was drenched in her tears. I had never seen my mother being so emotional, and I began to realize the gravity of my parting. I would not be seeing my Aai Dada for a long time. The distance would be too vast and expensive to cross. I left *Narayan Niwas*, my birthplace, with a heavy heart, eyes dripping uncontrollably. I was not even slightly aware that this pain of separation from my motherland would go so deep down within me, wounding my heart forever.

I had been on a plane only once before. Those days it was not so common to travel by plane. Dada and I started climbing the ladder one step at a time, holding Dada's hand as if I were still his little girl. When the air hostess closed the heavy glass door between us, Dada stood on the scaffold outside looking helplessly at me, while I lingered inside, unable to touch him. My Aaji told me later that after sending me off so far away Dada did not talk to anybody, not even Aai, for three whole days.

I was about to sit down next to Madhukar, when he jumped with a jolt, "Jyoti where are our chest X-rays?" He saw the passenger in the next isle carrying a huge yellow envelope in his hands. Those days, we were required to have chest X-rays declaring us free of Tuberculosis in order to enter America. Our X-rays had been carefully stored on top of a tall steel cupboard in our home at Dadar, so they wouldn't get wrinkled. Out of sight, out of mind; we forgot to bring them with us. For a moment we both sat stunned. It was the end of our journey before we even began. I ran to the air hostess and explained the grave situation to her. I could see Dada on the last few steps of the ladder which was attached to the plane. I could easily have run to him to tell him, or the captain could have sent a message to him, but she did not budge, and the door remained closed.

When Madhukar realized that our plane was going to stop for fuel in Karachi, Pakistan, we decided to phone Dada and ask him to send it to our final stopover before reaching New York. But when we reached Karachi, we were told that communication to the enemy country was not allowed.

Dada had lots of faith in astrology, and he made sure that all his three children would match their horoscopes to their spouses. He used to often consult his trustworthy friend who was a fortuneteller and an expert astrologer before he started on some new project or if he was facing difficulties in life. This time was no different. He had gone to his friend to ask for an auspicious day for our journey abroad. After all his darling little girl was traveling to such a long distance. Madhukar and I were very saddened to witness that in spite of Dada's efforts that our journey did not start on the right tune. We assured each other not to think negatively.

"*Pori* have faith in the Goddess, and she will always guide you to the right path," Dada's constant advice kept ringing in my ears. Dada's close friend was a travel agent. In those days there were no bargains or discounts for air travel and there were also no direct flights to America from India. So he had planned our trip rather cleverly. He got us on flights that would not make the connecting flights on the same day that we landed in the various European cities. In those days, the airlines would provide their stranded passengers lodging and boarding in a hotel; the airlines took pride in treating their customers to famous hotels in order to lure them.

Our first stop was in Beirut, Lebanon. I lost myself when I saw the beautiful peacock blue fan of waves in the Mediterranean. I had never seen such deep turquoise color in the ocean; the Arabian sea on Dadar's coast was always greenish gray. I fell completely in love with Beirut. We felt like royals while entering Hotel Phoenicia; indeed, it had originally been a palace. On the front steps stood a tall and stout Arabian man dressed in long *patlone* and *khamis* as if Aladdin himself had come alive. He was holding a gold tray with little golden cups in his hands. I felt a little timid of his daring black eyes and face full of beard and mustache. He came closer to me and handed over to me one of the cups. I was pleasantly surprised by his smiling gesture. He again gestured, and obediently I drank whatever was in the cup. It was the most bitter coffee I had ever tasted, despite its being flavored with cardamom. This was our first introduction to Lebanese hospitality. As we went inside the hotel, Madhukar saw Sabina Airline's office across the corridor and immediately had a clever idea. Our last flight from Brussels to NY was on Sabina. He explained the x-ray situation to the gentleman at the counter. The agent immediately asked, "Oh, if you would like, our man can go pick those papers for you." We both were surprised by his helpful suggestion. "Good Service to our customer is our only joy and goal' – I had seen this kind of slogan in the bazaar in Dadar, but to experience it in real life, I had to cross the ocean all the way to Lebanon. We were thrilled to have our problem solved so easily. With no more worries, we set out to explore Beirut full of gusto. After walking for hours we came across a farmer's market. Mesmerized by the abundance of vegetables and fruits - I had never seen such huge cauliflowers and watermelons - I thought I was in Alice's Wonderland. I was sad to leave Beirut so soon.

Next day our stay was in Athens, Greece. There was a coup just a few days before and armed soldiers were visible everywhere. We could feel the fear in the people and my heart was full of patriotic pride for peaceful, democratic India. As we were crossing the street, a man came running to me, "Are you Nargis, the famous Indian film star?" adoringly looking at me. For a moment, I was smitten with his admiration. But then I felt compelled to admit my true identity. The same thing happened when we were in the hotel. The gentleman at the restaurant presented me with a silver brooch. In a short while the truth came to light. Raj Kapoor movies were immensely popular here, and the Greeks adored his leading lady film star Nargis. Most of them had never seen any other Indian girl in a sari except on the silver screen.

The following day we gathered our luggage and flew to Zurich, Switzerland. It was exciting to see snow covered peaks of mountains. Until then I had seen Alps only in movies. I was eager to see them up close, so Madhukar took me to the nearby ski resort in a gondola. The enchanting view from my warm plane froze me as soon as we landed at the top of the mountain. My teeth started chattering with the severely bitter cold. Madhukar came to my rescue with a unique prescription. He handed me a very tiny glass of Drambuie and with a solemn face said, "Drink this *tirtha (blessed nectar)*. Bottoms up! It will wash all your sins away and your shivers will be gone."

I was such a gullible *pativrata* to follow my husband's command; I drank the liquid from the glass in a split second. The hot steam fired through my ears making me warm finally. It was getting late, and I was starving. For the last two days I had been deprived my simple everyday meal of *dal bhath, dahi, and roti.* Being strictly vegetarian, not even eggs were allowed in Aai's kitchen back home. I could not stand the distinct odor of olive oil rather than the peanut oil I was used to. After we inquired somebody told us about a local Indian restaurant. I was so desperate for my comfort food that I did not mind a long walk in the cold. Finally a heavenly aroma lured us to the right place. I wanted to order everything on the menu until I saw the footnote 'If you want *pakoras*, then we need 24 hours' notice'. Alas, our plane was leaving the next day, for our invasion of the Queen's Empire.

At Heathrow Airport in London, there were planes taking off every few minutes to anywhere in the world, so our trick of missing connecting flights didn't work. As we were dragging our luggage toward the taxi stand, I came across *Panjabi* women cleaning and sweeping the bathrooms at the airport. My privilege of being an Indian woman in a sari for the last few days was washed away instantly. Still, I was glad to see some Indian faces.

My cousin Suresh Bhagavat, Shanta Maushi's son, was studying in London. He came to receive us at the airport. As soon as we were on London's streets, I felt like I was back in Bombay again. But instead of being happy, I resented the *gora sahib*'s reign. My pride in our beautiful Bombay architecture evaporated as I realized that it was just a copy of London. All the buildings resembled my favorite Victoria Terminus in Bombay. London's gloomy depressive weather stung me more and all my enthusiasm vanished away. We were going to stay with Suresh in his studio apartment - no more Queen's hospitality at our service. Forget about the luxurious limousines or fancy hotels. All we had in our pocket was $14, a generous allowance from the Indian Government. So we used the famous Tube rail for the next few days. That's where we saw lots of hippie culture. I could never figure if a person was a man or a woman with their strange long hairstyles.

So far, our journey was really delightful. We were on our way to Brussels, our last stop in Europe. We both were silently worried about our chest x-rays, but as soon as we arrived at the airport, there was an announcement, "Mr. and Mrs. Joshi please come to the Sabina counter." We jumped like children, clapped our hands, and hugged each other with joy. At last we had the precious X-rays in our hands.

Once again, we were honored guests of Sabina Airline, and another palace turned into a hotel was our abode. "I could get used to this lifestyle very easily," I whispered in Madhukar's ears. Remembering a small dressing mirror at our Dadar four room apartment where nobody even had their own bedrooms, I was a little embarrassed, looking at multi replicas of myself in the mirrored walls of the luxurious bathroom. Madhukar feasted on a scrumptious meal as the chef came and cooked his culinary expertise of fresh fish at our table. '*Hay Kambkha tune pi nahi*'- So much to drink but you haven't even taken a sip. The cook was saddened that I could not do justice to his specialties. I asked him sheepishly if he could make me plain white rice? Within moments, white rice arrived in a silver fancy dish. We decided to make the most of our last stop before starting our 'real life' and headed to explore the city next morning. I was astonished to see a flower bazaar in the middle of the harsh cold winter. That was the first time I saw the miracle of a greenhouse.

Our 10-day European honeymoon ended too soon, and we took our final flight to discover Columbus' America. I was getting really tired of being confined in the airplane seats -like a golden cage again.

***

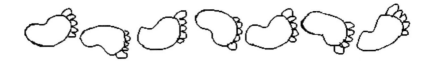

November 13, 1967

We were surprised by the custom officer's pleasant smile at LaGuardia airport in New York. He did not even open our bags. We took a small plane just 12 seats for our concluding destination to Decatur, Illinois. To get to this new land of my dreams we had traveled across 6 countries and 3 continents in 10 days! Our final airplane ride to the new world, but today I was too exhausted to enjoy it thoroughly.

The gray sky was hovering over the town. It was only 3 p.m. yet the sun had already set, and a light snow started falling. I was so weary that I could not fully appreciate the warm welcome of the gentle snowflakes caressing me.

Dr. Eicker, Madhukar's new boss, came personally to receive us at Decatur's airport. It was so small, I thought Pune's bus stand was bigger! After his formal but friendly welcome and shaking of hands with us, he abruptly asked Madhukar, "So Dr. Joshi, tell my why exactly you are here?" His straightforward question totally shook me off my feet. *What did he mean? After 9 long months waiting, after he had asked the Illinois senator to get Madhukar here as soon as possible because the newly developed Advanced Mental Institute of Adolf Meyer Zone needed him?! At last we were here, and he was questioning our arrival? Was he going to tell us to do an about-turn?* Madhukar, his faced composed, calmly answered with a smile, "Well, I have some special knowledge that will be valuable to your project, Dr. Eicker. I liked what you offered me in your letter. So I am ready to give you my full expertise. I am ready to work with you. That is why we came across the continents." Dr. Eicker thumped Madhukar's back cheerfully. "Yes, we will make a good team." His full-hearted laughter melted all my fears away. The official relationship of boss and employee would eventually turn into a genuine friendship. I was in awe to this introduction of honest American life!

***

Dr. Eicker had booked us into the local five-star hotel that night. I met a few people inside the hotel; they all looked same to me with their blue eyes, blond hair, and white golden skin. I could not make out who was John and who was David, who was Pam and who was Diane. I could not understand a word of what they were saying, their Midwestern accents so different from the British English I had learned in school. I didn't see a single person on the streets, only fancy cars scurrying along the spotless roads.

The beautiful hotel room, TV, all this could not charm me. Unknown language, strange faces, odd-smelling food. The odor of bacon at breakfast took all my hunger away. I was brought up in a joint family and our house was always packed full of people. Here there was not a single Indian person to be seen! So far away from Aai Dada. Homesickness piercing continuously. For the first time in my life, I felt isolated and lonely.

I started crying hysterically that night, "Raja, I don't want to stay here. I don't like your America. Send me home to India, first thing in the morning!"

"Jyoti, naturally you are very tired from this long journey. You are suffering from jet lag, which will make you depressed. Stay for a while. If you still don't like it here, we will go back. Don't worry," Madhukar tried to comfort me. For him this was not new. He had spent five years in America, when he was studying in Cleveland. I felt a little assured by his firm promise. I pushed away emotional Jyoti and decided to give a sincere try to live in this new world.

Next day we went to the bank to open an account. The bank manager took us out for lunch, to show their appreciation for a new client. This was a total surprise to me, having been used to long queues in our bank in Dadar. We would have to wait in the line, a metal tag with a number dangling in our hands, to be called upon by a bank clerk with a very blank expression stamped on his face as if he was doing us a favor. After lunch, the manager even helped us to find a studio flat. It was a little outside of town and quite small, but we decided to rent it because it was furnished and very close to Madhukar's office. That very same evening the manager came with us to buy a secondhand car, so casually, as if we were just going to the market to buy some fresh fruits. Luckily Madhukar got his driving license without any problem.

That night we moved into our very own new flat. It was inconceivable to me to get a new apartment, car, and bank account in just one day. I dreamt all night that I was in a *Maya Nagari*[4]. The next morning Madhukar left for his new job at 8 a.m., promising me that he will come for lunch around 12. I was happy to see at least the sun was out. The bright rays made me forget my jet lag and I decided to go for a walk. I didn't feel like putting on all the armor to fight nasty winter temps, so I stepped out of the apartment just to feel the weather. The sunshine was very deceiving. The bitter cold weather stung my skin. I turned to go back inside but just then with a loud thud the howling wind slammed the apartment door in my face. I tried to turn the doorknob, but it was locked. I was not used to the concept of carrying house keys. In Dadar our door was never locked unless we were out of town. Next door, the Garde family, we always had each other's key. In Dombivali, Madhukar's parents were always home. I rang the bell next door, but nobody was home. The thought of staying out in the veranda made me shiver even more. Not a soul was in sight. The apartment manager's office was at the other end of our complex. There was no way I could walk there in my house slippers and a night gown. I would have to wait until Madhukar returned for lunch. I started meditating to keep my mind calm. I became aware that I needed to be self-reliant. From that day on I always tied the house keys on my sari's *pallu* like a Bengali bride.

We were tired of restaurant food. So the next day Madhukar drove me to the grocery store. Once again, I was astonished by all the abundance. Fruits, vegetables, and other food neatly arranged in an eye-appealing manner to tempt customers. We did not have these large stores in Mumbai. We had our grocer at the corner, the

---

[4] Mayanagari – the city of May was named after Maya the great ancient king of the asuras. He was known for his brilliant architecture. In *Mahabharatha*,

vegetable vendor and banana peddler at the footpath in Dadar. If only I could bring them here to see this bountiful paradise. My feet lingered at every item in the aisles. I was overwhelmed to see limitless packages of sugar, flour, rice and so much more. When I left India, there was still rationing of food. The Indian government generously gave every household 500 grams of sugar and flour for the Diwali celebrations. I timidly asked Madhukar, "How much sugar I can buy?"

He smiled, "Jyoti you can buy as much as you want. Nobody will stop you!" We did not own a lot of material objects in the Dadar flat. Under the abundance of Aai Dada's affection I never felt the need for them. But now seeing the rich standard of living, tears started rolling down from my eyes, spoiling the sweetness of the 5 lb. pound bag of sugar in my hands.

***

Within a week we were able to move to a larger one-bedroom flat in a complex with a club house, swimming pool, and tennis court. That flat was equipped with a dishwasher, oven, stove, hot water, washer, and dryer. I had all the modern conveniences at my disposal. As soon as we emptied the two grocery bags, we realized we still needed dishes, pots and pans, and utensils, etc. So the following week was busy with shopping. I felt like a little girl again playing dollhouse.

When I left India there was no television in Bombay. When the TV was delivered to our flat, I couldn't really understand the language, but watching all the commercials helped me identify the products I would be buying in the next shopping spree. The whole day went by while I was glued to the screen until Madhukar came home in the evening. I confessed that I had not even taken the time to cook anything. I was afraid of his disapproval but my darling husband, car keys dangling on his fingers, took me out to a nice restaurant in town that evening without a single complaint.

I decided to make up for yesterday's laziness. I planned a real feast for my Raja. I was brought up in a Brahmin family and our diet was strictly vegetarian. Deciding to be daring, I bought steak to surprise him. I figured if it takes so long to cook potatoes, it must take longer for meat. I turned the oven on and put the steak in an hour before he would arrive home from the office. He was pleased seeing the table set, "What's so special today, flowers and all this?"

As soon as he sat at the table, I served him the steak right from the oven. He took a lot longer than usual to finish the dinner. Then he calmly said, "Jyoti next time when you want to cook steak for me, I will show you how to broil it in the oven, it takes only a few minutes." "Oh my God, did I turn it into a piece of leather? No wonder you were chewing it for so long! Raja, why didn't you say anything? You really didn't have to eat it," I shuddered with guilt. Holding my shoulders, looking into my eyes, he whispered, "I was admiring your courage. I know it must have been hard for you to handle that piece of meat. I did not have the heart to tell you." I melted in his embrace, thanking him endlessly.

Madhukar used to leave very early in the morning to go to office. I did not have a driver's license yet, so my whole day would be spent at home being lonely without seeing anybody. I was brought up in a joint family. My five maternal uncles or my aunt Aka's four sisters and brother were part of our family too. There was always somebody visiting us, ending up staying for dinner. So I was never home alone. The four walls started closing in on me. There was knee-high deep snow on the ground, but it was still a sunny day. I decided to go for a walk. On top of my sari, I put on a long sweater, a winter jacket, a scarf, and a cap to cover my ears. I made doubly sure the keys were in my pocket and went out. The chill air still made my teeth shiver, but I was going to conquer the road under my heavy boots. There were some houses along the roadside but still not a single soul on the road. All of a sudden, a dog came running after me. Having been bitten by a dog in my childhood, I was afraid of the dogs. So I started walking faster but another dog came to join me from the house ahead. I was petrified by their vicious barking. I began to run. Every house must have a dog, and they all came after me. I turned back and ran for my life toward home. The snow piles made it difficult to run and I was panting out of breath when I finally reached home determined not to go on that road ever again.

So instead I started walking on a two-way road going towards Madhukar's office. But now the cars on the road exchanged the role with dogs and were beeping at me. Many times the drivers would stop and offer me a ride. I tried to assure them that I really was just going for a walk and they would eye me with a puzzled look, *you must have escaped from Adolf Meyer-the mental hospital.* People were not used to see anybody just strolling. Later some people from Madhukar's office scolded him for not letting me have a car.

Once Madhukar and I went for a walk in the evening. I was wearing a white sari. Light snowflakes started falling. Catching the gentle flakes on my face I began to glide with joy. There was a little girl at the window, her nose rubbing against the glass. She came trotting outside towards me, "Are you an angel?" Nobody had ever given me such a beautiful *kitab.* "Maybe," I replied, hoping it was true.

One morning I was trying to get the home in order. The doorbell startled me. Somebody visiting me. Who could it be? I really had not met anybody except some clerks at the grocery store. I was so happy that I almost ran to the door. A blond haired, blue-eyed doll was standing at my threshold. I was a little taken back, as I didn't know her, but I sure was excited to see her smile and her extended hands. "I am Judy. I live next door. I saw you moved in the other day, so I dropped by to welcome you. Please take this, I made a watermelon peel pickle." *I chuckled silently to myself; back at home, we fed watermelon peels and other scraps to the goats and cows.*

Almost a week had gone by without really having come across any American person with whom to have a conversation. I was stunned. I could not imagine an American woman as a housewife! I had only seen her in big sunglasses, high heels, mini skirt flirting with the hero in Hollywood movies. I was thrilled to meet Judy. She christened me with a new name similar to hers: Jodi. She started taking me all around town and she helped me a lot to settle down to the American way of life. When I entered her apartment, I was shocked to see all the indulgent items there. I thought they were very rich but found out that her husband was a postman.

Our postman from Dadar appeared in my mind, walking sluggishly in the scorching humid Bombay heat, worn-out *chappals* on his feet, a heavy khaki bag on his shoulder, overloaded with letters and parcels, sheepishly asking for Diwali *baksheesh* from us.

I soon realized that American people were not shallow and materialistic at all. They were friendly, honest and hard working. I thoroughly enjoyed their company. Unknowingly I also began to enjoy the luxurious lifestyle. But as soon as I lay in the bed at night all the people back home sleeping on the foot paths, hungry children begging, would appear in my dreams. *"Everybody is born according to their karma"* – the teachings of Bhagwat Gita. I kept gently reminding myself not to spoil the golden present.

I decided to visit the YMCA, it was the day they were celebrating International Women's Day. Seeing me in a sari, the photographer hauled me into the group of other ladies. Next day that photo appeared on the front page of the local newspaper! Instant fame. I started taking tennis and bridge lessons at the Y, hoping to meet some friends. When I told Madhukar about the huge swimming pool at YMCA, he insisted that I should learn swimming. At the same time in the middle of winter I started taking driving lessons. So began the crash course in American life. I was getting tired of washing my saris every day so Madhukar suggested to try a new attire of Western clothes.

I decided to please him. I have come a long way. I remember that evening very vividly. I had come home from college wearing a *Punjabi* dress that my friend had insisted I should try hers. I was very pleased to see my reflection in the mirror on the wall. So I thought I would wear it home and surprise everybody. As soon as Dada came home from the office, his harsh voice shrilled in my ears painfully, "What is this nonsense? Take that dress off immediately. Girls from decent families don't wear that kind of dress." My mind was charred. I wanted to shout back at him, "My friend wears them, and she comes from a very prestigious family." But I could never backtalk to my father. My hair was always tied in a single braid, I had to wear bangles, my forehead was always adorned with a red kunku dot and my body covered in a sari. These were Dada's strict rules which I as a daughter had to obey.

To pay 60 rupees for an hour for the driving lesson was too much. I was still constantly converting dollars into rupees. But the instructor was really friendly, and he was very curious about me. I was still the only sari-wearing creature in Decatur. He was very chatty, asking me so many questions about India. Somebody to talk to every day was good for my loneliness. I looked forward to his interview every day. Soon I got my license. The car wheels became my wings. I was free at last to go where I pleased.

My friend Barbara invited me to go to her club. They were having a fashion show. I was the least interested in the latest styles, but I happily accepted her offer. Isolation was suffocating me. I could not live without friends. I needed to be with people. I was very touched by the affection and friendship I received from everybody at the club. There Barbara introduced me to a minister's wife. I was quite impressed with her. She was kind and down to earth. No trace of her husband's status. We had a heart-to-heart chat, and I got invited to her house for tea. I couldn't wait to go home and report to Madhukar about my invitation to a minister's home. "Jyoti, he is not a government minister like in India. He is a church padre," Madhukar tongue-in-cheek, popped my balloon. I was not familiar with colloquial language, but soon enough American English vocabulary started swarming in my brain: A lift was *an elevator,* a drinking tap was *a fountain,* taxi was *a cab,* and a dickie was *a car trunk.*

I started teaching once in a while as a substitute art teacher in the public schools. Our principal would eat his lunch at the same table with the custodian. This was an especially important lesson to me, to experience fairness and to see this society treat people equally. I was proud to be a part of the community. Whenever I met somebody on the street, I was always greeted with a smile, a simple sincere greeting, "Hi, how are you? Have a nice day." I felt at home. I joined their pilgrimage full heartedly.

Soon it was going to be *Kojagiri*, the autumn full moon festival. The taste of Kesar-flavored sweet milk was still lingering on my lips. I decided to invite a few friends from our apartment complex to celebrate. I was puzzled by everybody asking me about attire. "Oh, we usually wear white on that night," I replied without knowing the hilarious scenarios that would come out of it. This was the first time

I was having guests. I got the apartment ready and wore my favorite special white georgette sari with glittering sparkles. Madhukar also wore his white *Lakhanvi embroidered Kurta*. The doorbell rang. Sue was a nurse at Madhukar's office, and she came wearing her starched white uniform. Then came Katie in her pure white bridal gown! Her husband Garry was wearing a plain white shirt and khaki pants. Michael wore colorful clothes, confessing while pointing at his white tennis shoes, "Jyoti this is the only white I could find." Henry whistled at us as he entered the house in white shorts, smiling mischievously while he took off his white baseball cap and bowed. Madhukar's camera kept clicking. The entire group looked so funny, filling our apartment with continuous laughter all night. They loved my spicy *bhel* and *keshari* milk so much that they all went home with a doggy bag – a new concept to me. Madhukar had driven me to the only Indian grocery store around, 60 miles away in the Champagne-Urbana university town to buy all the ingredients for bhel.

I was humming *Tarana*[5] of sweet bonds of friendship, feeling comfortable in Decatur among our newfound friends. Two years swiftly glided by the new horizon. The girl who wanted to go back to India as soon as she landed started sprouting happily in this foreign soil.

Helen, my angel, appeared in my life coincidentally. She was interviewing me at an employment exchange office. She was rather surprised to hear my story. Those days a girl from a foreign country coming to America was not common. She invited me to play ping pong the same evening at her house. She could not find me a suitable job, but she made plenty of room for me in her affectionate heart. The mere seedling of acquaintance blossomed in a shady tree of deep attachment and friendship. Madhukar and I became an inseparable part of her family. Every holiday we would be celebrating at her table. When I was expecting, she gave me a surprise baby shower and she wrote to my Aai not to worry about her daughter. Aai was relieved that Helen was going to look after me after the baby's birth. I found my *Maher* at Helen's.

---

[5] Tarana, a Persian word meaning a song, is a type of composition in Hindustani classical vocal music.

Our daughter Swati was growing faster than the moon phases. She was almost 6 months old. Suddenly Dr. Eicker got a huge grant from the NIH and we were going to be transferred to Boston.

Nonchalantly in my youth I left India. I thought I was ready to take on a voyage anywhere in the world, not aware of all the potholes on the road ahead. I was heartbroken to leave my loved ones then but survived the exodus. Roots of new friendships in Decatur burrowed deep in this foreign soil. I was not aware that the pain of separation would pierce me again every time I would move to a new place.

It was easy to find happiness here only because of the wisdom imparted from Aai Dada and because of Madhukar's constant gusto. I thought I had the ownership of all my accomplishments! What a fool I was. It was they who invested in me. I realized this only when I went so far away from them. I am in their debt forever. Not a day passes without remembering my parents. Dada's strict discipline side-by-side with his funny sayings and affectionate pampering, Aai's delicious cooking and wisdom. I became well aware of the secret behind my successful journey so far.

***

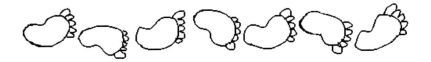

October 10, 1969

My motherland is many moons and miles behind me…
But I have carried carefully,
In my hands, this gift of Sanskar.[6]
My country changed but this earth remains tranquil.
I have become attached to this earth.
I unfolded my tent here of my own free will.
These many years entangled in all my friendships.
Behind my mask, there is still one gypsy wandering …
And wondering, "Who knows where the next stop is?"
An echo pounding in my ears,
"The whole universe is my home."
Yet, when Diwali celebration comes, and
The little panti[7] flickers on my backyard fence,
So do the memories on my mind's screen.
Thoughts of my friendships' reflections overwhelm
And there is a big tidal wave of memories
In the oasis of my wandering soul!

Leaving all our newly found friends that made me feel at home in Decatur behind … Carrying our precious 6 months old Swati-a small U-Haul stuffed with all our belongings we hauled away 1200 miles, all the way to Boston.

I have never seen Autumn so beautiful. Winding roads, tall maples bursting with orange, yellow, red, and brown standing in a parade to salute us with colorful carpets of leaves. I lost myself in *Rang Panchami*. Madhukar and I knew right away that our decision to come Boston was the right one!

---

[6] The heritage/culture you carry with you from your parents and surrounding.

[7] An earthen lamp with oil and wick

I had never heard of the strict rules of housing before. Most of the decent apartments in Boston did not allow children which was very maddening. We felt compelled to buy a house in spite of our empty pockets. We bought a small house on a pond in Framingham. The night we moved in the house, both of us were tossing and turning...tormented by the idea of such a large amount of loan, from the bank. We were not used to American way of borrowing. We could not sleep. Nobody we knew in India had owned the house at such a young age. Having your own house in old age was a lifelong dream.

Dr. Eicker's grant from the NIH was associated with famous Brandeis University. So Madhukar started his new job as a professor at the Heller School in Brandeis. Opportunity for abundant education and world-renowned universities - Boston was quite similar to Pune in India. As much as the people were very liberal and progressive, at the same time they were extremely traditional old style as Pune's educated *Brahmins* society. In fact, I was amused to hear the term 'Boston Brahmins'.

Soon I found out that it was very difficult to break the ice in first introduction with Bostonians...I was used to the friendly Midwesterners in Decatur. Luckily, our next-door neighbors Linda and David were friendly. Linda was from Virginia. They had three boys who were a little older than Swati. Linda was very fond of girls and soon our children started playing together.

Madhukar was enjoying his job. Our small world began to blossom in the cosmopolitan city of Boston. Soon we found lots of Indian cultural activities around us. I was thrilled to see few Indian families in Framingham, especially when I bumped into Manda and Shaila, two wonderful women who were from Bombay and spoke *Marathi*, my native language. That was the beginning of lifelong friendship.

I got involved in a newcomer's club. Subbing in the public schools helped me to meet more people and started making few friends in town. Three years went by very quickly and our family grew with Chitra's birth.

I became a mother for eternity, busy taking care of my two darling daughters. Still, deep down in my heart, it was not enough. So when

Chitra started preschool, I decided to volunteer at her school. It opened a new door for me. In a few days I found that I had been given a special skill to teach young ones, and I took courses in early childhood education. When both girls were in elementary school, I became a pre-K teacher full-time. It was a perfect job for me; I could be home when the girls were home. I developed my own curriculum, using art as a medium with which to teach language, math, and science skills. When our director Janet saw the success of my teaching methods, she encouraged me to enter a competition for art projects. I won 1st prize and my projects were published by Gryphon House in a craft encyclopedia. I started giving workshops for parents and teachers. My students' parents were quite pleased with the outcome, and I became their favorite teacher, so much so that if the younger siblings weren't put in my class too, the mother would start crying. Yet in truth I knew that the real teachers were my innocent little students.

Meanwhile, I also started teaching yoga in the evenings. Those yoga classes were well liked by people, so I started giving more classes in the neighboring towns. I had finally found my niche.

I never dreamed I would be a yoga teacher. It began when we started taking our girls to the *Vishwa Hindu Parishad* camps. At the camp we met a *Shastri, a* learned scholar, who needed a place to stay for a few days. So naturally we opened our doors to him. While he stayed with us, we found out that he was an expert in yoga practice. I always wanted to learn the asanas but never had the chance to pursue it in India. So Madhukar and I became his students. At that time, yoga was just starting to become popular in mainstream America. After a week of lessons, he told us to teach others. Yet we really did not feel confident in our knowledge or skill.

At the same time, Madhukar's career progress came to a sudden halt because of university politics around tenure. Up until that point he had been rapidly climbing the ladder. I tried in vain to convince him that with his excellent achievements he would soon find another suitable job without any problem. But he could not take the emotional blow and became very depressed and felt desperate. That was the time when the Shastri had arrived in our home; he instantly picked up on Madhukar's vulnerability and pounced. He started by giving

Madhukar a *Mantra* and promising that it would soon shower him in gold; of course, in return he wanted money from us as a fee. I was alarmed by the Shastri's behavior. Mantras are sacred and are to be given by a worthy Guru to improve one's spirituality, and not for material gains. I was shocked to see my husband, who normally would not buy into this kind of scam, fall prey to the Shastri's maneuvers. I tried to convince Madhukar, but he would not listen. After putting up with this for a while, I finally told him, "You have to make a choice. Either the Shastri goes, or I go." I was so relieved when Madhukar realized his mistake! Despite this, we did actually start teaching yoga and I owe our success in this venture to the Shastri's advice.

Soon I decided to go beyond the physical asanas and started studying the philosophy of yoga and meditation on my own. I grew up in a very pious household and there would be always some kind of worship ceremony going on in our house. My parents would go listen to pravachanas (discourses) on *Vedanta* philosophy in the temple. They used to urge me to join them, but I was too busy playing with my friends as a 9-year-old girl would be. One of my 8th grade teachers taught us to recite the 15th chapter of the Bhagavad Gita by heart. I am afraid that was just *popat panchi*- parrot's mimicry; the deep meaning of the stanzas did not penetrate my heart. In my final year of high school, on a whim I accompanied Dada to Swami Chinamayananda's lecture on the Gita in Shivaji Park. I was completely transfixed by the Swamiji's command of Vedanta philosophy and the eloquence of his language. I went for the entire week of his lectures.

Kelkar Maushi, Aai's close friend and well-known leader of *Rastriya Seva Samiti*, the Indian Women's Service Association, used to give pravachanas on the Ramayana. For the first time, listening attentively to her, I utterly understood Sita's power and strong personality. Kelkar Maushi planted a seed of woman's liberation in me. Although my Aai always thought independently and did not blindly follow traditions, I only recognized this when I was far away from her. Later while I was in college, Malu Maushi, Aai's childhood friend, was a follower of Ramakrishna Paramhansa and she also gave discourses on his life. I was so impressed by her style that I actually skipped the collage and attended it all. I was lucky to hear J.

K. Krishnamurthy's unique ideology in a beautiful surrounding of our J. J. College of Arts. I became deeply interested in Indian philosophy and was pulled to Yoga. But I never took time to learn any asanas while I was in India. My mother would always remind me to do Sun salutations. I was a typical teenager and always found excuses.

Our house in Framingham was very blessed by Swamini Pavitraji and Swami Parthasarathy. Not only that, but lots of famous books on Indian philosophy were delivered to our doorstep without our asking. Madhukar and I were extremely happy with these boons. One such incidence occurred when Mr. Sharad Godbole, a founding member of the *Brihan Maharashtra Foundation*, was on the phone. We did not know him personally but had heard of him. He read one of my articles, '*Achieve Shanti through yoga techniques'* in a BMM magazine about stress management. He came to visit us, and as soon as he entered the house, he opened his bag and poured all 52 tapes of *Vimalaji Thakar's* lectures onto our dining table! Then on every evening we would listen to her lectures.

***

On my yoga students' request I decided to do a whole day retreat. I was very excited for the first session at our house. Our home would be filled with Om vibrations. But the day dawned with a dark shadow on my face. I felt funny and could not open my right eye. When I looked in the mirror, I saw right cheek drooping down, and I felt numbness on that side of my face. I decided to ignore my crooked face and continue with the yoga retreat. According to all the participants it turned out to be a great success.

Next day after some tests, my doctor announced it was Bell's palsy and I started taking medicine accordingly. But the whole week was extremely excruciating and there was no sign of improvement. My face was still crooked. I was mortified. Madhukar was busy in his office and the girls with their school. Nobody had time to pay attention to my face. Though Madhukar became extremely quiet, which I knew was the sign of his worries. He would often draw into himself in under stress, with no communication at all. If I got sick, he would bring or suggest all kind of remedies for me but would have hard time consoling me with comforting words. That was his nature. I should have been used to it by now, but I still felt neglected. I was scared my face would never get back to normal, having heard of cases like that.

The eye refuses to close,
hitting a heavy lid on my courage.
ears longed to hear the breath of life.
I could not find the music.
Taste ruined by tongue.
Hungry for one affectionate glance from you.
At this very moment when I need you the most
you lock yourself inside stony silence
and start building the iron walls that defeat my strength all together.
You disappear beyond my horizon, piercing me by your muteness.
Where are you, my Raja?

Luckily, my face became normal in a few weeks.

***

One day I merely said if only my parents could see this country. Immediately Madhukar fulfilled my dream to have Aai Dada at our home abroad. He invited them full heartedly by sending airline tickets. I could not wait to see them crossing our threshold. Chitra was only 19 months old, and Swati almost 3 years. Dada had just retired. He was about 60 and Aai was 54 years old, but I thought they were ancient. This was their first trip out of India. Their enthusiasm was overflowing. Swati and Chitra both were spoiled by Aaji and Ajoba's pampering. Aai could not speak or understand much English, but somehow managed to communicate with all my friends. My father, who would frown at us if we were going to a Bollywood movie, was now hooked on watching soap operas and the Watergate proceedings. He would often confess, "This would never have happened in our India!" He was amazed to witness the honesty and truthfulness of the senators' dedication to preserve democracy. "If I were 10 years younger, Jo, I would have settled down here very happily," Dada admitted to me one day. He loved America from the bottom of his heart. In fact he would often interrogate me, "Jo, why have you not become a U.S. citizen yet? Everybody's *janmabhumi* – land of one's birth and *karmabhumi* -

land of one's karma-action is different." But I was not yet ready to give up my motherland.

Madhukar had returned to India after his PhD. But during his job search there, in spite of a deep desire to help his motherland, Madhukar had a sour taste in his mouth because of all the big companies' bureaucracy. He missed the freedom he had experienced in the U.S., which resulted in his return to America. The love for our new country America was growing rapidly in both of us, and Madhukar had urged me many times in vain to become a citizen.

***

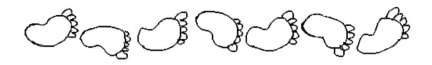

Sāre jahān se acchā, Hindositān hamārā Ham bulbulen hain is kī, yih gulsitān hamārā [8] *- Our Hindustan is better than the entire world, it is our garden, and we are its nightingales. - poet Muhammad Iqbal*

1976

Reading the Boston Globe while leisurely sipping hot tea was our favorite activity on Sunday mornings. The tranquil was shattered by loud noises from our backyard. We went to look out and were surprised to see all our neighbors gathered and applauding. On the picnic table sat a cake representing the American flag in red, blue, and white frosting. Linda was winking at me mischievously. I had forgotten that only yesterday I had mentioned to her during our daily chitchat, that Madhukar had newly become a citizen. We were both struck speechless by their warm gestures of friendship.

***

October 31, 1984

When Jyoti looked at the clock, it was exactly 9:20 in the morning. She decided to have her second cup of tea. The girls and her husband had left the house in the early morning as usual. She loved being alone on Mondays, her day off. She never watched TV in the

---

[8]An Ode to Hindustan is a patriotic song for children written by the poet Muhammad Iqbal. The poem was published on 16 August 1904. Publicly recited by poet Iqbal the following year at Government College, Lahore, British India (now in Pakistan). The popular song quickly became an anthem of opposition to the British Raj.

daytime, but today unwarily her fingers reached for the remote, intrigued by the famous actor on a talk show. Suddenly his interview stopped, "We interrupt this program for breaking news…" she heard the reporter's hurried announcement. "The prime minister of India, Mrs. Indira Gandhi, has been shot as she was walking from the garden *Raj Bhavan*, her headquarters for the press interview. One of her personal bodyguards assassinated her." Jyoti almost choked on her tea.

Indira Gandhi had previously declared a State of Emergency and all members of the opposition party, especially Jan Sangh's members, were put in the jail under her iron hands. Jyoti's Aai was a member of Samiti, the women's organization that supported Jan Sangh. All her uncles also used to attend Sangh meetings, as did Madhukar when he was in India. One of her uncles had been jailed by Indira Gandhi for his activities.

Jyoti had taken Swati and Chitra to India a few years back to show them the authentic way to celebrate *Diwali*. They were visiting a *Rangoli* exhibit, Jyoti on the 3rd floor and Swati on the 1st. Seeing a *Rangoli* portrait of Indira Gandhi, Swati shouted loudly to get her attention, "Aai look, that is Indira Gandhi, the woman who put your uncle in jail, right?" Listening to Swati's announcement, Jyoti felt so embarrassed that she wanted to bury herself. Her daughters were both bilingual from a very young age. She had taught them both to write and read Marathi. As most of the Americans could not understand Marathi, she would tell the girls that this was their 'secret' language as a way to entice and motivate them to learn. Swati had forgotten that she was in Dadar, where most people were native speakers of *Marathi*!

Yet despite her non-favoritism towards Mrs. Gandhi, Jyoti was sad to hear of the slaying. She became ashamed to be called a citizen of that India where this kind of brutal violence took place. Dada had constantly urged her during their last visit, "Jo, these days are not good, there is no return for you now. Gandhi's reign is ruthless. You should become an American citizen right away." She had been shocked to hear her patriotic father's advice. She remembered that conversation vividly now, and the decision was made instantly. That evening as soon as Madhukar came home from the office, before she could change her mind, she announced, "I am going to fill out the forms to become an American citizen."

***

Faneuil Hall, Boston – 1986

It was 10 o'clock in the morning when I entered Boston's Faneuil Hall. Just one more drop in the sea of people. Everywhere Korean, Vietnamese, European, Indian, white, black, yellow, brown, all colors were mixing in the melting pot. Everybody's face was stamped with unique emotions. Some were giggling, some were very solemn, and a few were a little shy. The man next to me had buried his face in the newspaper ever since I sat there. Not a single word. I wore a mask of aloofness. This cold attitude surprised me. When did I grow such a tough skin? There was no mutiny in my heart at all. I had been avoiding this moment for the last 19 years! Just the thought of giving up my Indian citizenship would evoke a fluttering tricolor Indian flag in my mind. Where had that proud Indian Jyoti gone? Today that same woman had come here to become a citizen of the United States. In a few moments all 38 years of being Indian would be shed like a snake's skin. As simple as cutting her fingernails! No pain, no hurt. Metamorphosis! A strange calm before the storm. My mind was numb. All that turmoil of emotions disappeared into the unknown.

"If the time came, would you take up arms against the enemy?" The question in our written test was still haunting me! I am a worshiper of non-violence, a follower of Gandhi! *"This whole universe is my home"*; the Vedic doctrine is embedded in me. There are no boundaries in my mind.

I left the sheltered home of my loving parents and came here as a newlywed bride of hardly 20. I was rebellious against the old Indian traditions! But something strange happened since I came to America - I discovered the value of Indian tradition, culture, and philosophy. I became more Indian here than I ever was in India. I wonder how this was going to change now that I was about to become an American Citizen? Would the official stamp on the paper change my inner core? "No!" my mind insisted. But that piece of paper still mattered. Without it I wouldn't be able to teach in public schools. I wouldn't find a proper job to earn my living.

"Everybody please rise," the judge finally arrived. The right hand was raised. The oath was repeated, *"To be honest and loyal to the United State of America."*

Sounds of claps like firecrackers burst everywhere. My mind was still absolutely quiet. They say, when a loved one dies, sometimes the person left behind does not cry. Her tears dry all of a sudden. I think that is what happened to me. At 2 p.m. in the afternoon I was a full-fledged American citizen, on paper. Funny! I didn't feel any different! I went back to school to teach the afternoon class.

"Congratulations Jyoti, I am glad you are one of us now!"

Everybody was telling me. I thought I always had been one of them. As soon as I stepped into the class, I was buried in shouts of "Surprise! Surprise!" Little boys and girls were dancing in a parade, waving American flags, singing *"This land is your land; this land is my land..."*

Mera juta hai Japani, Ye patloon Englistani, Serpe lal topi Rusi, Fir bhi dil hai Hindustani. - My shoes are from Japan, these trousers are from England, the red hat is from Russia, but my heart still belongs to India. This famous song from the movie Shree 420 started echoing in my heart.

Lightning crackled in my mind. In the midst of chaotic thoughts my mind went back 4 years ago to when I was visiting India. It was the 15th of August, India's Independence Day. I was at a traffic light. A little beggar girl was running in the maze of traffic, selling India's flags. At least one flag should be sold so she can buy some food. Before I knew it, I rolled down the window of my air-conditioned Impala and bought every single flag she had. My young daughters were carrying those flags so tenderly, as we boarded our returning flight to America. The flags are still proudly decorating the walls of my home.

"You're a grand old flag, you're a high-flying flag!"

The children were still singing happily. I came back to the present. Something was dripping on my cheeks; at last my tears were flowing freely. All these dear friends showering me with their - gifts, well-wishes, and love. They were celebrating for me. Can this little piece of paper turn the world so upside down? Aha! But that piece of paper would fatten my paycheck. Alas, after all, those dollar notes are also just pieces of paper!

***

1997

Motherhood! How I had carried the laurels of Motherhood so proudly! But lately its glory was disappearing from my body. I felt like bone-dry wood. At the same time I started suffering from allergies. These changes affected the contours of harmony in my mind. I began to sink into that turmoil. I was too emotional, sometimes crabby and depressed, making others miserable. I did not know how to get rid of it. I read every advice book and medical article I could find. In the end went to my gynecologist, and he suggested hormone therapy and some antidepressants. I refused to take either. The Surgeon General could not confirm that one of the side effects of menopause was depression. Madhukar and I could see a certain pattern – there were only certain days when I would become moody. So with his strong support, I decide to override the drugs.

Madhukar was overloaded with the growing responsibilities of his job. My darling daughters were away and very much involved in their careers. Nobody needed me anymore. I felt left out. Madhukar and I were alone in our empty nest. Borders Bookstore was our favorite hangout. We would inevitably purchase the latest books to take home with us. One Friday Madhukar ordered a nice gourmet coffee and sat reading a book on astronomy while I found my favorite, Rumi's poetry. After an hour or so, I came back and sat next to Madhukar. He was so absorbed in reading that he did not even notice me. After waiting a while, I poked him and asked, "Do you still remember me?" He questioned me back with a straight face, "Who are you?" That was his usual style, always teasing, but I took it to heart. I don't know what happened to me. I completely ignored the mischievous wink in his eyes and took it literally and felt very hurt. Without a word I furiously scratched something on his paper napkin and threw it at him.

You are the center of my universe.
Like earth circling to her Sun, I dance around you.
Yet you ask me, who am I?
Lingering in the aisles of the grocery store,
I look for the sugar contents of each item to control your diabetes.
As evening spreads its shadows,
I listen to your Camry's motor to start frying your favorite curry for dinner.
Your loving caresses, where have they gone?
In the loud thunder of a speeding subway
You used to hum poetry in my ears,
coming so close to me, cheek to cheek
But now you don't see the dark circles under my weary eyes!
Have you forgotten to harbor me in your heart?
'How was your day?" our mundane end-of-day exchange.
"Fine, fine," you murmur before immediately grabbing the remote to watch the evening news.
You wonder if the world is falling apart.
But inside these walls your soulmate is choking, and you don't even notice.
I am sinking in the sand of your aloofness.
I am searching for the oasis of your love.

He read it, folded it neatly and put it in his pocket without a word. I was about to lose my calm, but I saw him moving quietly closer to me. He held my hand in his hand, looked deep in my eyes, "Jyoti, how can you even doubt my love for you? You know how much I love you!"

***

I wished I could rip the days from the calendar. Each day was more agonizing to my moodiness. Hot flashes were unbearable on this scorching summer day.

"You want to go to the beach? It always makes you happy. Cool sea breeze and the ocean waves would soothe your body," Madhukar recommended a remedy. I nodded without a word and obediently sat in the car.

Gloucester beach was an hour and half away. The long car ride aggravated my back pain fiercely. I felt like a rotten tree covered with termites swallowing my *chi*. Madhukar put Vimalaji's sermons on tape and listening to her calm voice on therapeutic *Dnyaneshwari*[9] soothed me momentarily. The rhythm of the drive caused me to doze off until the wheels abruptly came to a halt. I woke up to a deep blue ribbon flowing; in front of me a gentle surf was whirling against a giant rock. I was puzzled. We had come to this beach so many times, but I had never seen this rock in the water before! It must be a low tide.

'Come! Merge in me!' the silent call from the Atlantic became loud in my ears. Ignoring its call, I chose to sit on the wet sand. The sunbathers were swarming at the beach, and yet I felt lonely and fatigued. My darling daughters' silhouettes appeared on the seashell's mica, seagulls carrying their giggles. If only they were here, definitely their hugs would have cheered me up. The waves resonated *Omkar*. My mind feebly tried to merge into *Dhyana* without success. Far away on the horizon there was a white sail- upon which I focused my vision. *Dharana*[10] had become only a meek action. The last two days the same chaotic crazy mind was ruling over me.
"I want to stretch my legs; I will be back in a while," Madhukar started walking.

I do not know how long I sat there. I was startled by the rough roar of tides. The huge waves started coming in rapidly over the rock making it disappear in front of me.

---

[9] The *Dnyaneshwari* - a commentary on the *Bhagavad Gita* written in Marathi by Dnyaneshwar- the teenaged saint and great poet.

[10] Dharana (Sanskrit) - focusing your mind on an object or thoughts in preparation for meditation.

"Oh, you are still dry? Let's go in," Madhukar's hand pulling me. I took a deep breath and immersed myself in the icy cold water. It made my pain numb and I began to enjoy it. *When did my strange fascination of the ocean start? Was I a fish in my last life? Did I get caught in the net! Was it my childhood on Dadar's beach?*

Suddenly the waves pulled me into the past … Zakir Hussein's palm impulsively striking the tabla, losing himself in *Nada*. The concert hall echoed with the beats. It was not just mere sound, it was *Nadbrahma*[11]. It pierced me beyond that sound shedding all my thoughts and pulled me into Dhyana …

Why couldn't I do the same now? I shut my eyes forcefully. If only I could find that Nadbrahma again*!* My mind became still momentarily, bouncing back and forth like a piece of driftwood at the shore. I could hear a tribal dance pulsating. Wait, did I hear drums?

My eyes wide opened. High tide was in full swing, lapping my body. I heard the drums again. Was I delirious? The pounding of the drums became loud and tangible. My head turned, and I saw in the distance, people of all different colors and ages dancing, gesturing their hands and feet in cadence. It was not a hallucination after all. My footsteps inevitably went towards the circle of dance. The drummers were almost in a trance.

Dha Dhin dha… Dha dhin dha [12]

Wrinkles of wisdom covering her face, the old *Babushka* whispered to me from the dancers, "Aren't you going to join our party?" I was a little intimidated by her graceful dance, and shook my head, confessing, "I can't dance like you." "Then how come your hands are swaying, hips are swinging, feet are tapping on the beat?" she smilingly pointed. "No, I don't belong to this group. I can't dance," I continued to protest. "Try at least, *dance as if nobody is looking,*" she winked at me again.

---

[11]Nadbramha (Sanskrit) - the sound that existed in the beginning; the sound and vibrations from which the universe was created.

[12] Dha Dhin- are the notes of tabla.

I realized that my mind started singing their tune, my body started dancing with them. The whirlpool of thoughts calmed down. Waves of rhythm flowed in my body. I became one with them; I was submerged into ecstasy.

The drummer pushed his drums towards me and without any hesitation I grabbed the drums and started beating lightly, the repressed primordial sound started to unfold...

I can hear the sound of Anahat [13]*.*
I do not need any lessons,
It was in me from the very beginning,
it's my birthright.
I am one with the sound.
This is the magic of Nadbrahma...

***

1980

I was listening to Erma Bombeck's interview on the car radio. I always felt as if she was watching my family closely and importing all the funny stories from us into her writings. The idea of suing her had crossed my mind. I decided to keep a diary of my own for the record.

I parked the car in the garage and started upstairs. "Mom, where is my bra?" Swati yelled out in her soprano voice! Our house echoed with these kinds of dialogues, my teenage daughters always accusing each other of stealing their clothes. Startled for a moment, I checked myself, thought *maybe I have it on*? Again Swati shouted, "Mom!" I was still in the basement and she was on the second floor. I shouted back to her "(next door neighbor) Linda borrowed it."

Balancing three grocery bags in my hands I climbed the stairs to the kitchen, out of breath. My darling husband was lying on the sofa in

---

[13] Anahata (Sanskrit)- unstruck, and unbeaten. Anahata Nad refers to the Vedic concept of the mystic sounds heard at the beginning of meditation.

his favorite yoga posture, *Sheshashahi Bhagawan*, Lord Vishnu lying down. For a split second I dream of our past life as newlyweds when he ready to please me at every minute.

"You must have gone to the grocery store," he said passively. Hearing his words I came back to reality.

My retort was lost in the racket of the football game, Madhukar's eyes glued to the screen. If Meg Ryan had walked into the room while the game was on, I guarantee he would not even notice. He would definitely win a contest against the sage who failed to control his temptation for Menaka [14] while attempting to meditate for supreme power!

I had the fear that if he ever found me lying dead on the floor, he would say, "Oh, she is dead, can't do anything now! So let me at least finish this game!"

I could hardly manage to put the bags on the counter before running to the bathroom. My hand reached for the toilet paper, but I couldn't squeeze the Charmin because only the empty cardboard roll was there. I calculated that I had changed the rolls twice a week in 3 bathrooms for the last 16 years, a staggering 4,992 rolls! I deserved to be in the Guinness Book of World Records for my efforts.

Some day when God is visiting me, I am going to ask her, "How come you made all the members of my family deaf, mute and blind?"

If once in a blue moon my dear husband had to go to the grocery store on his own, I had to give him a map of the aisles. I kept Xerox copies where I marked the location of bananas, milk, bread. As usual luck was never on my side, and the grocer would inevitably rearrange the items and Madhukar would come home defeated and almost empty-handed. He would be carrying ice cream, which he attested was the essential item of his diet.

---

[14] In Hindu mythology, Menaka is considered one of the most beautiful of the heavenly celestial nymph.

The other day it was raining. "Where is my umbrella?" he asked me accusingly, as if I had hidden it somewhere. He started his drill of looking everywhere – in the car, in the closets, in the house, without any success and went into despair as if he had lost something valuable. It is our usual routine: he would lose his watch, wallet, etc. and I, the *pativrata* (devoted wife) that I am, would locate the item in under a minute. We had six dining chairs, one for each evening of the week where he puts his jacket, when he gets home from work.

Once we had a dinner party, I tried to give him crash course in 'How to be a gracious host; Do not start eating before the guests have been served. Don't ask me loudly which item on the menu might not be enough.' These lessons never sunk in. When the guests arrived, I signaled him to offer them a drink. After much poking he went inside…

"Jyoti, where is the ice?" his loud words from the kitchen startled the guests in the living room. I counted to 10 and try to maintain my serenity with a forced smile. "Check the oven, I was baking them."

* * *

Many years have gone by since then. Our daughters are grown up and settled down successfully in their own lives. Our empty nest is too quiet. Today in my restless cleaning frenzy, I found my old diary. Those were the days, after becoming members of the Marriage Encounter group, that we wrote love letters to each other. This particular page unfolded in front of me.

You keep the drawer open, and I close it quietly.
When you forget to turn the light off, after leaving the room.
I immediately rush to turn it off.
You are always hot. I am always freezing.
So the cold war begins, our thermostat the battleground.
Your wet towel lands on our bed after you take a shower
and I silently hang it on the bar.
'Let's make tea."
Before your words dissolve, I obediently put a steaming cup of chai in your hand.
I make your favorite fish masala for dinner.

You gobble it up without saying a word of appreciation, lost in your science fiction book.
I want to watch TV, but the remote is in your hands.
The Sunday paper is scattered all over the house after you read it.
I iron the pages into neat folds before putting it in the recycle bin.
I am cooking a gastronomic meal the whole day.
You innocently wonder," Are we having guests tonight?"
I gently suggest, "The house needs to be vacuumed."
Why? You are so puzzled.
After much coaxing, you vacuum two rooms and declare your fatigue,
locking yourself in the bedroom for a nice nap.
The guests sit down for dinner, the table lit with candle lights adorned with my beautiful fresh flower arrangement.
You ask politely, "Did you all see Jyoti's flowers?" and efficiently move them and smiling with relief.
Turning the chandelier to full brightness, you exclaim with satisfaction,
"Good! Now we can all see each other without obstructed views."
I am a dutiful guard, keeping your diabetes in control
But somehow you manage to eat the Basen laddus.
I feel very romantic seeing the full moon peeping into our bedroom window.
You are engrossed in the book of astronomy, measuring the distance between the moon and the earth.
I am watching a funny movie on TV, while you are seriously solving math problems on the computer.
I go for my morning walks on the lake enjoying my retirement from teaching.
You just started consulting again after having retired for the third time.
You are eager to lock my creativity in the frame as soon as I show you my new painting.
You skip lunch, very busy with your business meeting.
I am busy in the company of famous artists in the museum and enjoying a leisurely luncheon with friends.
In the evening I come home, tired, wondering what to cook?
You read my mind; ready to save me, car keys dangling in your hands, you smile,
"Why don't I take you out for dinner?"

*All I said the other day was, "Our garden looks barren."
Immediately you took charge and the earth flourished with freshly planted flowers.
All the old scars, complaints, grumbles remain,
but now they echo with loving harmony.
I understand you truly.
We do make a good team! Really... a great team!
Your love is constantly flowing through my veins.*

I love you, Raja.

***

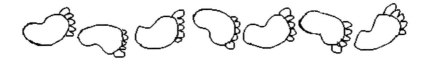

January 11, 1989

A long time ago my dear friend Ellen told me about the group that she attended. "Ellen, what does it mean?" I was confused by the title, 'Marriage Encounter (ME).'

"Jyoti, it teaches a couple how to communicate with each other and many other secrets of a successful marriage," she answered confidently. I will babysit your girls. Chitra and her Peggy were just toddlers. "Obviously, you do not know my husband', I murmured under my breath.

I love to take life-enrichment courses. Both of us had gone to *The Silva Mind Control* workshops before. So I decided to give it a try. That evening I told Madhukar about the ME weekends in Rhode Island, handing him the brochure. '*Restore communication. Heal conflicts. Reconnect with each other. Restore the romance*'. He did not want to go, just as I had expected. "When would you learn to communicate, then?" I tried to convince him to no avail. Finally, I gave up.

Many years went by. He had gone for a mandatory retreat weekend organized by Digital. When he returned, his confession shocked me, "Jyoti, from now on I am really going to listen to you. I thought I was taking your class! Please tell Ellen that we want to attend ME." Hallelujah, there was light at the end of the tunnel after all. I offered sweets to my goddess, thanking her profoundly. Ellen and Dean had since moved to Buffalo, New York. The girls were away at college. So without much ado we were on our way to the retreat.

In the introduction the speaker warned us, "If your relationship is not in harmony, this is not for you. It is not counseling." But then he guaranteed that when we leave the place, the ties of our loving bonds would be tighter than ever. This mathematician husband of mine was not known to verbalize his love for me. The first session was all about how to ask questions to your spouse. The technique included holding each other's hand and opening the conversation with something positive about your spouse. I was worried that Madhukar grabbing my hand might escape suddenly. We were given specific topics: *What are your expectations of each other? Which behavior of mine hurts you the most? How can I improve our relations?* It was a long list.

I was surprised when Madhukar asked me a question while looking deeply into my eyes. After 22 years the soft touch of his palms still sent a loving wave to my body.

Na Bhuto Na Bhavishyati- there never was nor will there be… Was this really happening? His eyes were almost teary, he was so emotional! He started reading the questions to me. We were an old married couple by that time. Supposedly we should have known all the answers by then. The sessions went all day with only a brief lunch break. Lots of serious topics were handled, questions that we would never even think of or dared to ask. It was an intensely intimate experience. We were witnessing the intricate layers of our love and the threads of our companionship were knitted strongly together. In the endearment workshops we were told to write love letters every day. In doing so we found the valuable hidden gift of our everlasting love for each other. It turned out to be a little honeymoon after all. Then the party began, and we were married again in Jewish style, under a canopy. We were emotionally exhausted by the end of the weekend but I was convinced that the divorce rate would go down drastically if the government made this workshop mandatory. The next day, on our anniversary, my diary became eager to dialog…

Raja, your super speed train is going same time on many different tracks.
It has only two compartments- one for your office and other for your two princesses.
Oh, my beloved please don't rush like this. I see a red signal ahead.
Wait at the station for a rest.
See your queen is waiting for you.

***

The ME organization helped us to create a group of five couples; we started meeting monthly at each other's houses. Our cultural backgrounds, professions, and ages were wide ranging. Ian and Shira, a young newlywed couple, had moved here temporarily from Israel. They used to live on a Kibbutz. Jack, a senator of Massachusetts, was eighty-five years young, and had been married to Eileen for 45 years. Judy and Ernie were our group leaders. Lesley was a musician and her husband David a scientist; they were from Rhode Island. Every time we met; a host would organize the meeting structure. We would prepare one answer to a question at home and would be given one question on the spot during the meeting. Then our letters and the answers would be discussed openly. The group became very close. I used to love our heart-to-heart talks. I would take time and write an answer, while Madhukar, at the last minute just before we would leave for the meeting, would scratch something in his notebook. I used to console myself that at least he is coming to the meetings full heartedly. Once when the meeting was at our house, I greeted our friends with one of my favorite Bollywood movie songs, with the melodious voices of Geeta Dutt and Hemant Kumar.

'Nahi chand hoga na tare rahenge...Magar ham hamesha tumhare rahenge!
Perhaps the moon or stars might not be there, but I will always be yours forever!

Next question was, 'If you were not in this world, how would I cope'? I do not know why I choose this particular topic to discuss. Was it a premonition of the future? We wrote letters and then discussed the answers with our spouses. After so many years, I found a sweet secret! My absent-minded professor could actually write very romantically. I saved all his letters, holding so near to my heart, for eternity.

***

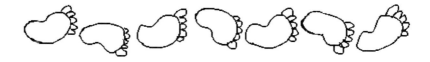

June 1, 1987

Swati's graduation and my niece Tanuja's wedding were both in June, so it was a perfect excuse for Aai, Dada, and Akka to visit us for the 3rd time in Framingham. There was a huge snowstorm on the day of their arrival in May, very unusual weather for that time of year. I knew it wasn't going to last long, so I prayed to Mother nature to keep the snow on the ground until they reached our home. They had never seen snow in person having lived in Mumbai all of their lives. It was sheer joy for me to watch when they began to jump in the snow and throw snowballs at each other like little kids.

Madhukar was going to officiate Tanuja's wedding in Chicago. We were all excited about this *muhurta*, the very first wedding of this new generation. The preparation of this gala was in full speed.

My usual daybreak rush was no more since Aai took over the kitchen as soon as she came. We were enjoying her delicious, spicy stuffed eggplants and *Gulab jamun* marinated in sweet rose syrup. It was eight o'clock in the morning and I was on my way to school, delighted that I would be reaching work early, as I liked to catch a little extra time before my students arrived. I put the morning chanting on in the car. But as I approached the signal, even though it was green, the traffic was at a standstill. I craned my neck to see what the matter was. An ambulance went by, followed by a shrieking fire truck and a frenzied police car. I clenched the steering wheel, and muttered with frustration, 'No such luck to reach school early today'.

As soon as I reached my classroom, Janet, our director, came hurriedly to find me, "Jyoti, there is a phone call for you." Who would call me so early in the morning? My girls must have forgotten something. I went into her office and picked up the receiver.
"Are you Mrs. Joshi, Madhukar's wife?"
"Yes, I am, why?" I was puzzled.

"I am calling from the emergency room at Framingham Union Hospital. He has been in a car accident," the aloof tone of her voice sent a chill through my body.
"Oh my God, is he alright? Please tell me he is ok?" I crumpled onto the chair, frantically impatient to hear her assurance.
"Sorry, according to the rules of the hospital, I am not in the position to tell you."
Trembling I told Janet. I was on my way to the hospital.

As I rushed to the hospital, I kept telling myself to calm down and not be so creative in my negative thinking. I wanted to reach the hospital safely. I tried to concentrate on my breathing.

Bureaucracy was holding me at the entrance. I hurriedly signed all the forms, and only then would the receptionist tell me that a drunk driver had collided with Madhukar's car, which was totaled. My heartbeat skipped at her words. I ran toward his room.

Madhukar laid down in the bed like a wounded prey, his eyes closed. But I could see he was alive! A deep sigh of relief flew out of my mouth; I hadn't even realized that I was holding my breath. His face was black and blue, and his right eyebrow was bruised. But his eyes were safe, thank God. I reached forward and gently kissed his forehead. He looked at me.

All the courage that I had gathered until now melted and I started wailing, holding his hand, "How are you, my Raja? You must be in lot of pain, how can that idiot drunk do this to you, what happened??"

"I am ok, Jyoti, but honestly, all I remember is I heard the siren and then I saw a giant machine ... that's all, nothing more."

"Oh, my god! That sounds like they used the 'jaws of life' to extract you from the car!" My mind went numb.

"Jyoti, I could hear that stupid woman talking to you on the phone. I yelled from the room, let me talk to my wife so she won't panic. But she completely ignored me. What kind of a #%$ nurse is she? Acting more like a prison guard."

Listening to Madhukar's colorful language, I was convinced that my dear husband was alive and well, and I thanked goddess Mahalashkmi profoundly.

In a few minutes, a doctor entered the room. He told me that Madhukar's right kneecap was crushed completely, and he would need to be operated on right away. I was frightened of immediate surgery. "Doctor, I would like a second opinion." The words slipped through my mouth. He firmly answered, "You are entitled to do that but then you won't be able to save his knee for sure. There is no time to waste." I did not know this doctor at all, how could I allow him to cut into my husband just like that? I poured out all my doubts about his credentials in a very humble tone.

"Please forgive me doctor, I have lot of questions about this surgery. I don't know anything about you or your success rate in this type of surgery." He smiled and calmly declared, "Of course, I truly understand. Shoot all your doubts at me. I will try my best to answer them." I listened to him for a length of time: He had been a practicing surgeon for a long time, and he lived on Flanagan Drive, the road familiar to me as some of my friends lived there. I felt kind of a momentary relief but was not ready to decide right that moment. He left the room for me to think it over in private. I had forgotten to ask him about the recovery time, so I ran after him. In the corridor I saw our dear friend Dr. Rohit Janghi hurriedly walking towards another room. In my chaotic mindset, I had totally forgotten that Rohit worked at the same hospital. I was thrilled to see him, and without thinking I yelled to get his attention. I purposely asked him in Marathi, "Rohit, do you know this surgeon? He wants to operate on Madhukar in an emergency. Please, I need your advice." After listening to the whole saga, Rohit assured me calmly, "Jyoti, I've known Dr. Bard for a long time. He is a very good surgeon and I trust his judgement. Go ahead without any fear, let him do the surgery." I was so relieved to hear his confidence. Rohit was like a younger brother to me. He walked with me to see Madhukar and stayed with us until it was time for Madhukar to be transferred to the O.R.

"Why wait here? We don't know how long it will take. You go home, I will call you personally after it is done." Dr. Bard promised me as he went after Madhukar. Then Rohit gave me a friendly pat on my back and said, "Jyoti I will be there in the surgery room with him." I told Madhukar that he was in good hands. God has sent us two angels today. I took Madhukar's briefcase and left the hospital reluctantly.

"Jyoti, how come you came so early today, and what is this? You are carrying Madhukar's bag?" Aai's sharp gaze caught the briefcase in my hands. I collapsed on the couch and started sobbing. Aai came rushing followed by Dada and Akka. I hugged them as if my life depended on it. Tried helplessly to narrate the incident, "Aai, Dada, Akka, I strongly believe, Madhukar is alive, he was saved, because of your blessings, your presence in this home!" Every morning our porch would be full of vibrations from their spiritual chanting. The next four hours were the slowest ever, as if the clock had frozen. Dr. Bard did call after the surgery as promised. Madhukar was still groggy when we saw him in the recovery room. I thanked Goddess Mahalaxmi again and again for her *krupa*.

All the festive planning dissolved. Swati's graduation party was canceled. Such a strong girl. I did not see any trace of disappointment on her face. She was cracking jokes as usual and making us laugh. Underneath her bubbly personality there was such maturity. I am so blessed with my two darling daughters. With a heavy heart we had to tell Tanuja not only that her uncle wouldn't be officiating her wedding, but he wouldn't be able to attend at all. It was decided that except us two, everybody would go as planned. The surgeon had warned us that the recovery would be very painful and slow, "His leg has to get used to not having a knee cap."

When I returned to the school, I found out from my colleague Doris, whose house was on the hill where the accident happened, that she saw the accident occur and called the ambulance. The same ambulance which made me late going to school, was carrying Madhukar to the hospital. Her husband was a police officer, and he ran down and helped supervise. But they did not know it was my husband they were helping. They became his angels at that atrocious moment. Next day I took a basket full of long stem red roses to show our gratitude, which she would not accept at all. She graciously said, "We are glad that we were there to help." The world is full of wonderful souls. I told her that I would pay her kindness forward always. From that day onwards, whenever I see an ambulance or fire truck, I always send out a silent prayer.

As Madhukar was discharged from the hospital, Dr. Bard told Madhukar seriously, "You can almost do anything except two things. You won't be able to play football and you won't be able to kick your wife anymore," and then he let out a big peal of laughter.
"Oh, thank you, thank you so much, Dr. Bard, for rescuing me!" I joined in his laughter.

Madhukar had to start walking after only a few weeks according to Dr. Bard's orders. Even though he used crutches the pain was excruciating, and he would try to hide the tears in his eyes. Seeing him in that condition, Dada was overwhelmed with compassion. He loved Madhukar like his own son. He started giving him a gentle massage with herbal oil. That was Dada's specialty. He had learned the technique from one of his constables. It helped Madhukar tremendously. Pretty soon he started walking on our street holding my hand. It was only ¼ of a mile, but it would take him almost half an hour. He did not give up. We would walk every day. I convinced him to wear a *lungi*; it was more practical than pants. It took him almost six months to start walking normally. We met an Indian doctor who was a renowned knee specialist. He claimed that Madhukar would never be able to sit down on the floor ever again. I knew my husband. He would never give up but would accept the challenge. Aai's uncle Babuji Dandekar from California showed Madhukar how to do certain helpful yoga asanas. Madhukar's motto in life was always '*Never flinch, never turn your back to the problem, face it and find the solution always!*' So he followed Babuji's advice in spite of the pain. He started practicing the postures day and night and defied the negative prediction!

***

July 10, 2012

I needed to find some important papers, so I was searching upstairs in Madhukar's office. I came across a rare hidden treasure - some of Madhukar's old letters. One of them was written to Dada. He loved my father as his own. He used to tease me that the only reason he married me was because I was Dada's daughter! There was a special bond between them.

I remembered Madhukar telling me about the very first time he met Dada. "When he was in my office, suggesting a marriage proposal for his daughter, I was quite impressed by his good heart and sincerity, in spite of working in the [corrupt] police department. Honesty was deeply etched on his face. So I decided if she is his daughter, I must look into it."

Later when we were newlyweds, Madhukar told me, "Look at your parent's loving relationship. If we can achieve that in our marriage, Jyoti, we will have a happy life together."

I wonder how in the world Madhukar knew Aai Dada's secret in just one week. Madhukar had an extraordinary talent of seeing to the core of a person at glance of first meeting. My Dada was indeed a *jaganmitra*, friend to the universe! He would conquer your heart the moment you met him.

***

November 1989

All four of us had planned a special trip to India in December to celebrate Dada's 81st birthday. There is a prayer ritual called '*sahastra chandra darshan*', which means 'the seeing of 1000 full moons.' We had just celebrated Thanksgiving at our house. The next early dawn, I was awakened by the phone ringing. The sky was still dark, and groggily I answered the phone. It was Aba, my brother, calling from India. My heart skipped a beat! Why was he calling us this early?

"Jyoti let me talk to Madhukar," his voice was quivering.
"No, Aba, talk to me, what is the matter? Why did you call?"
"Dada is no more." His words froze my mind.
I felt guilty that I was not there with him at his last moment...

'Jivet sharada shatam', *'may he live to see one hundred autumns.'* The prayer vanished before it was even spoken. The world would never be beautiful again without my Dada. Just two days ago he came to visit me in a very strange way. I was wide awake, but it seemed like a dream. I could feel his being right next to me. His visit lasted only for a minute, but it was very real.

His loving memories crowded my mind like a starry night. I jolted out of bed, ran from the second floor skipping a few steps at a time, to make a foray in the garage. In a frenzy I started digging through the garbage can, my bare fingers raking for his letter that came last week. How could I have thrown it away?! At last I found it and started reading it fanatically over and over again. It would be his last letter, his everlasting relic to me. When I first came to America, I used to write letters to him. It was a slow process but cheaper than a phone call. He would reply back praising my style, encouraging me to write all the time. I think that's how my writing habit developed. His constant advice to me was, "When in Rome, behave like the Romans." My traditional father, who had not approved my fashions while I was living under his roof, started admiring my western clothing.

Precious memories started falling, like a broken string of pearls, all the pearls tumbling one by one. His smiling face appeared before me, a smear of red *Kumkum* between his eyebrows, pure white delicate cotton shirt and dhoti, that was his attire around the house.

Sometimes a special car would take Dada to his office at the police headquarters, next to my college. But he would not allow me to ride with him. No special treatment. His ethics were very high. He would move heaven and earth for anyone who needed his help. There was always somebody at our house asking his advice. They would bring him a box of *mithai,* or a basket of fruits, but he never accepted these gifts, which he considered bribes. We were also strictly under obligation not to accept anything while he was not home. I was always disappointed and only understood the significance when I was much older. He would say, "Never sell yourself for any favors. The minute you put a price on your service, your value becomes zero!" After he retired, a lot of his friends in higher positions wanted him to join their companies, tempting him with a rich salary. But my father refused all the offers, telling them, "Today you are my dear friend but if I start working for you, then you will be my boss, and I will be your servant." Dada's colleagues would feel a little inhibited by his strict discipline. But the people who knew him well would see that behind the stern expression on his face, there was always a little gentle mischievous spark hidden in his eyes.

I almost did not recognize him in photos from his youth, his head was covered with thick black hair! Ever since I can remember, Dada was bald. He would spend a lot of time in front of the little mirror combing the few strands of hair that remained. I would tease him, "Dada, there is nothing on top of your head, why even bother?" He would wink at me and say, "Jo, it takes a lot of skill to part four delicate hairs!"
He would come home in the late evening from office in humid and sticky weather. We could not afford a fan or air conditioner. Dada's back would be covered with heat rash. After dinner I had the boring job of scratching his back. Reading my mind, he once said, "Pori, how can I explain the affection I feel through your touch? When you rub my back, it feels like my Aai has come back to life."

Then I would feel very guilty. He had been orphaned at the tender age of 8 years when his parents died in the worldwide 1918 flu epidemic. Shyam, as he was affectionately called by his mother, took his baby brother under his wing. Dada's maternal uncle took them to live under his roof despite having his own family of eight children and a wife to support on his paltry teacher's salary. Shyam left his uncle's house after high school and started living on his own in Pune. He wanted to go to college but could not afford it, so instead he moved to Bombay as a young lad of only 19 years to earn his living. In the end Dada established himself successfully and did well for his family.

Now I felt like an orphan without him. My heart longed to hear his lullaby '*Pandurang Hari, Vasudeva Hari*'. He used to sing his favorite bhajan to me every night while massaging my legs. I was not truly aware of our meager financial situation until I was in my last year of high school. There was a constant air of joy and contentment when I was around him, I had always thought I was a millionaire's daughter. We did not have the material objects of comfort like a refrigerator or even a fan, but there was never a shortage of warmth and love in our home. Dada never indulged in buying fancy things for himself, but he was very generous when it came to his children's wellbeing. Then his motto would be 'k*hain tar tupashi nahitar rahin upashi', I will only eat food covered in ghee or else I would rather starve.* He never went for cheap stuff for us and would always buy the best quality goods even if it cost a lot of money.

Dada pampered me with beautiful silk saris. Every time I would wear the sari he bought me, a black Kanjiwarm silk with orange border, one of my favorites also, he would admiringly say, "Jo, you look like a princess!" But if I lingered in front of the mirror getting ready to go to college, he would scold me, "You should pay more attention to the beauty of the heart than of the flesh." I grew up listening to all his proverbs and sayings. I accompanied him on his early morning walks. The sky would still be sleepy. He would stop by his friend's yard for some Prajakta flowers for *puja*. Under the tree the earth would be festooned in a carpet of those celestial flowers. He would bend down and start collecting them, while murmuring morning stotras. Without a direct doctrine he taught me an appreciation for *Parmeshwar,* God Almighty. I climbed the very first step of *bhakti, the devotional path*, by his example.

Every Sunday was cleaning day for him. Our apartment would be spic and span. He loved to go to the market to buy fresh vegetables and fruits, especially on festival days when we had big celebrations with our extended family and friends. He would join Aai laboring to shell the *Dalimbya*[15] and to wash the banana leaves which we used instead of paper plates. *'No job is too small!' 'Pay attention to whatever you are doing and take pride in it. Achieve the best results-Yoga karmasu Kaushalam-when you put your heart into any action that is the real yoga'-* I learned this philosophy from his everyday habits. His ritual was to do *puja* and *Arti* every morning after bathing. At *Ganesh Chaturthi*, the *'Ganpati Atharv shirshya'* jap would echo in our house for hours. He would chant the *Devi Mantra* one thousand times during the Navratri celebrations at Mahalakshmi temple. Our porch vibrated with his *mantras* and invocations.

---

[15] Dalimbya, a dry bean delicacy in Kokan, Maharshtra where he came from, is also known as Birdya or Valachi Usal. Soaking the beans few days and shelling it one by one by hand is a very tedious process. Val beans have exceptional nutritional values.

Dada and I were out for an evening stroll. Just the day before we had celebrated his 76th birthday in our enclosed porch in Framingham. As we were walking, he stopped abruptly, looking at the affluent houses in the neighborhood, "Pori, forgive me that I could not build a house like my colleagues did. I did not give you and your brothers much." My hand reached over to close his mouth. "'Dada, what are you talking about? That is absolute nonsense. You have given us a *Kalpvriksha*[16]. Your teachings, your lifestyle, your actions are our most valuable treasure." He told me constantly that this was going to be his last visit to America, which I refused to believe. Unfortunately, his intuition came true.

Dada used to frequent a local restaurant in Bombay, where he met my mother's maternal uncle Appa. Appa Uncle was quite impressed with this bright young chap. He had a favorite niece Kamal (my mother) who was 17. He strongly urged my grandfather to propose his daughter's hand to Shyam.

Without seeing each other beforehand (that was normal back then) Shyam and Kamal got married. The *barat, wedding procession*, was about to begin when it started raining. So instead of a horse carriage, the newlyweds walked under one umbrella to the *Parshuram* temple in Chipalun. This is how their journey of life together began.

At the end, Ai and Dada were in a car on route to a neighbor's daughter's wedding when suddenly Dada became ill. Looking at his vital signs my mother knew this was not a normal sickness. She asked the driver to turn back right away. She did not want to disturb the joyous occasion. It had started raining and she opened an umbrella and helped him out of the car. Holding his hand, she slowly walked toward my Uncle Tatya Mama's house, which was on the ground floor. Dada collapsed as he entered the house. They ended their journey together under an umbrella.

As if a seam on a sack of rice rips open, scattering the grains around, all my memories of Dada spilled out of my heart on the

---

[16] Kalpavriksha, is a wish-fulfilling divine tree in Hindu mythology.

morning of sad news of his demise. These memories are like a thousand branches of *Vatvruksha.*[17] I will always cherish living under their cool shade.

Dearest Dada, I salute your immortal teachings and memories! Our family is flourishing today because of your hard work, vision, and constant support to give your children and brother the educational opportunities that you didn't have. We all owe everything to you.

I gathered myself and robotically got ready to go to work. Dada would have told me to do the same.

***

---

[17]Vatvruksha Is also known as Akshay Vat, the indestructible banyan tree, is a sacred fig tree mentioned in the Hindu mythology.

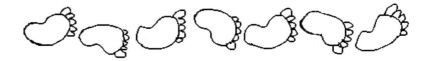

January 12, 1992

Time was rolling like a river. Today was our 25th anniversary. Our loving companionship, started with a few strands of colorful silk threads, now has woven into a shawl. I was awake next to him, he turned over and whispered in my ears, "Do you know what today is?"

"You remembered…The spark of your intelligence that blinded me, 25 years ago is still sparkling. Your enthusiasm rising every day like a sun…Your ever-green laughter blowing with a wind speed. I salute your gusto again and again,"

We were attending an Indian wedding in Newton, MA. The priest officiated the wedding by *Vedic*[18] tradition and explained all the of *Sanskrit* mantras and vows to the couple. Madhukar was sitting in the front row and I was in the corner with some of my girlfriends. This was the first time I was hearing the poetry and romance in the Hindu wedding ceremony. I was in awe! I found Madhukar's gaze fixed on me. My eyes filled with tears of joy. Twenty-four years ago, he and I had taken the same vows in Sanskrit but hadn't known what we were saying then. These wedding vows are four thousand years old, but the meaning can still be applied to modern times.

I murmured back in his ears.
"*Raja*, I pray the goddess to let our journey endure the next seven lives together. Raja, listen, let's do the saptapadi vows again on this day. When we got married, the priest was chanting them in Sanskrit, we really did not pay attention to the meaning of the words."

---

[18] Vedic philosophy, which shaped Hinduism.

"Yes, dear, you know that's what I always say to you." Listening to his words was music to my ears.

It took us three hours to reach 'Cathedral of the Pines' in New Hampshire, one of my favorite places. It's a memorial dedicated to all Americans who have served this country. I loved to just sit and meditate in the outdoor sanctuary surrounded by tall trees and paths full of flowers, with a gorgeous view of Mount Monadnock. We had gone there many times. This was a perfect place to renew our vows. I told the girls we would have 'F.F.F.' (forced family fun). The wintery weather was vicious, and the forecast said it was going to be record breaking abnormally cold (-12°F!). That didn't stop us though; we piled on layers of long johns, woolen pants, sweaters, winter jackets, scarves, and ski masks, and headed out. The parking lot was empty. Who else would be as crazy as us to come here in the middle of January! As soon as we got out of the car the bells from the tower began to ring; the vibrations echoing around us. I smiled to the girls, "Listen, it is a good omen!"

"Aai, it is 12 o'clock, that's why the bells are ringing." My daughter Chitra, an accountant, was being logical as usual. One time we were listening to a famous Hindi song, '*Jhan Jhan Payal Baje. Kaise Jau Pike Milanko? —My anklet bells are ringing so loudly, how can I go to my beloved? Everybody will hear them and know that I am going*'...Chitra taking all the poetic romance away, simply shook her head and questioned- why didn't the girl simply just take her anklets off her feet?

Snowflakes sprinkled gently like Jasmine flowers on our path. We started taking our seven steps, saying our vows, fully aware this time of what we were promising:

"Let us take the first step to provide for our household a nourishing and pure diet, avoiding those foods injurious to healthy living.

Let us take the second step to develop physical, mental, and spiritual powers.

Let us take the third step to increase our wealth by righteous means.

Let us take the fourth step to acquire knowledge, happiness, and harmony by mutual love and trust.

Let us take the fifth step so that we are blessed with strong, virtuous, and heroic children.

Let us take the sixth step for self-restraint and longevity.

Finally, let us take the seventh step and be true companions and remain lifelong partners."

I had always wanted a 'love' marriage. Finally I married my chosen mate.

***

Life happens while we are busy making other plans. - Unknown

December 1999

The millennium dawned with many changes in store for us.

Madhukar had developed many statistical formulas while working at Digital. He was always respected and honored by his colleagues. But mismanagement in the upper levels of the company resulted in the eventual unimaginable shut down of the giant company. Everybody was forced to either resign or move to the future buyer's company. Madhukar decided not work for a large company anymore. Some people from Digital got together and formed a small company in Merrimack, New Hampshire, and they wanted Madhukar in their close-knit circle.

After the profound enjoyment of living in Framingham for the past 32 years, we had to move our home base across the border. The strong bond of friends was hard to leave behind, but Madhukar did not want a long commute anymore. We found a beautiful home on a little hill in Nashua close to Madhukar's office. A survey by a well-known magazine had just concluded that Nashua was the best city to live in the United States. We fell in love with that *vastu*, blessed with constant sunshine and gently flowing wind. I christened our house 'Windsong'. We could see our beloved Mt. Monadnock from our second story bedroom on a clear day.

***

September 11, 2001 - Nashua, NH

Only fate knew that today's letter would be entirely different...

Ever since Dada passed away, Aai had been living alone in their Pune condo. It had been my ritual for the past 15 years to write her a letter every Tuesday. I started the letter with my usual traditional 'Shree', which wishes the recipient prosperity of each kind, not just monetary. But today that Shree was shattered by an evil mind. Full of frustration I crumpled many unfinished letters and tossed them in the waste basket ...

Earlier that morning I had finished my daily walk by the river and returned to the parking lot, my mind still humming like bees over the water lilies. Mahler's symphony on the radio pleased my ears. The lilies and music were enough for the day's muse. My daily ritual. But suddenly the music was interrupted by an urgent announcement, *"The World Trade Center in NYC has just been hit by a small plane!"* The news made me very irritated. "Nobody does their job with mindfulness nowadays. Especially the tower control peoples. Lately so many innocent people have died in plane accidents from sheer negligence," I grumbled.

As I neared home, there was another announcement, "This was not an accident but apparently is a terrorist attack! It was not a small plane but a regular passenger jet!" I could not believe what I had just heard. Somehow, I managed to park the car in the garage and stormed into the house. Car keys flopped on the coffee table instead of their regular hook behind the door. I even forgot to remove my shoes per tradition before I hurriedly clicked the remote. I could not comprehend what I was witnessing on the TV screen. The World Trade Center tower was an inferno. Then there was a second plane coming toward it. All the turmoil felt like watching a James Bond movie, but in an instant the towers broke into pieces and fell to the ground. It was not after all a Hollywood movie, but grim reality. I became numb.

The plane dashed through that burning tower in NYC, but it exploded a volcano in me, 400 miles away. People were running everywhere, just as my mind went wild without any direction. The terrorists attacked the tower, crushing it down with thousands of innocent victims whose suffering made my heart bleed. I was suffocating together with the people who had inhaled so much smoke and debris. I started looking helplessly for some remedy. How can I save them? What can I do to ease their pain? All these futile questions rushed to my mind. The assault was far away but still I felt as if my safe abode was being attacked.

The house went silent in spite of the loud screams on TV. The whole world was mourning and condemning this inhumane and violent act. America was brought to a sudden halt. In the middle of this chaos all the airports were immediately closed. I knew how hard and difficult task it must have been to do this in a matter of minutes. I remembered how Dada used to spend days on the phone organizing the traffic control in Mumbai when dignitaries were arriving for an official visit to the city.

I longed to be near my darling daughters. I called Madhukar but couldn't reach him, having forgotten that he was in an important meeting. I wondered if he even knew yet. I couldn't reach Swati in Worcester either, but was able to get Chitra on the phone at her office in Boston. As soon as Chitra heard my voice, we both started sobbing. The fragility of life slashed at me sharply.

I liked my peaceful home and had always enjoyed my solitude but today it felt like the isolation had frozen me. I needed human contact to thaw my senses. I called our next-door neighbor David, a pilot himself, hoping he could educate me on how this could happen, but his answering machine came on. I went outside. The street was deserted as most of our neighbors worked during the day. So I went across and rang Emily's doorbell. Emily, 80 years young, opened the door, a novel in her hand and reading glasses on her forehead. I knew that she had no idea of the catastrophe. I felt compelled to tell her yet at the same time regretted being the one to give her bad news like this in her old age. Emily was quite shaken up and I tried to comfort her with a cup of tea with no success. After Emily lay down for a nap, I returned home in a daze. I did not want to be in an empty house and wished Madhukar would come home early.

It was almost lunchtime, but I had no appetite; only my thirst for answers grew and grew. I sat in front of the TV motionless, hungry only for more of the day's news. When I had first arrived in America forty-four years ago, I was fascinated by the news programs, seeing the reporters actually at the scenes giving eyewitness accounts. That developed into a habit of watching the daily newscast with David Brinkley and Tom Brokaw. I remembered the way that the news of bombings during the Vietnam war had similarly traumatized me. All the shattered bodies of innocent Vietnamese people were still alive in a strange way, right in our living room with the help of our new color TV. *Siddhartha* of my mind slept in the comfort of worldly possessions within the safety of our four walls.

Each picture on TV was adding more bad news. The Pentagon was attacked. A fourth airplane went down in Pennsylvania. In only an hour this vast land was put on hold. There was nothing but turmoil in sight. This was not just an assault on a tower or land, but on individual freedom.

I felt that my usual phrase to end a letter *"With Love, Peace, and Joy"* was wiped away by the blood stains of the victims. A fierce rage was ignited, and my usual compassion evaporated.

Badala! Revenge!

Today I truly understood the destruction in Hiroshima and Nagasaki! To destroy this *Mahishasoor*[1], we needed *Mardini*[2] *to return*. I retreated into the mythological story my *Aaji* used to tell me. The pages from my school's history books fluttered. All the text of atrocity, the brutality of partition, the battles constantly waging in Lebanon. *History repeats itself!* The inferno in my mind was growing. My compassion seemed to be demolished. All I could think was an eye for an eye! This feeling was very unfamiliar to me. I never knew this brutality even existed in me, and it made me scared. I was ashamed of this new Jyoti. "No, no! This is wrong," I assured myself by saying it aloud. This is not righteous thinking. Only peace will win. But how do I find it? My heart ached for an instant solution. It will take ages to bring that peace to the world. *Sambhavami Yuge - When there is chaos and destruction in the world, he is born!* The famous stanza from the *Bhagavat Geeta* resonated in my mind. I called for the goddess, *when will you appear?* Isn't this enough destruction?

The day was wasted in restless feelings. It was soon established that middle eastern terrorists were behind this attack. People started reacting by taking the law into their own hands. They did not know any better, so all Muslims were put in the same mold, and misplaced revenge and violence ensued. Every *Sikh* who wore a turban was assumed to be Muslim. I remembered how I was called Muslim when I wore a *Khamis* and *Salwar*. I too was guilty many times of not recognizing the differences between Chinese, Korean or Vietnamese people; they all looked the same to me.

I wanted to help but did not know how? I was searching for an answer aimlessly. Suddenly like a flash of lightning, a new friend peaked through my clouded mind. I vividly remembered when I first met him. Scorching heat was fuming on that summer afternoon. Radio and TV newscasters were begging people to stay inside in during the heat wave. But I did not have that luxury, too many things on my day's to-do list. I saw the sign 'full service' at the corner of the road. I was tempted, rare in these days of high gas prices. The car automatically stopped there. The guy at the station came out to pump the gas. I could tell from his clothes and his face that he was *desi*, and I could not resist my curiosity, "Which part of India are you from?" He smiled almost in apology, "I am not from Hindustan." I immediately realized he was Pakistani and tried to correct my mistake. "It doesn't matter. After all we are all one, that is what I believe. "I wasn't sure how he would respond, but his positive answer made me happy, "*Bilkul sahi*... Absolutely true. But tell me, sister, why are you out in this heat? Please come in so I can offer you some cool *Mangola*." I was touched by his hospitality. His *Hindi* was sweeter to my ears than Mangola. From then on it had been our unwritten rule only to go to his gas station.

Finally, Madhukar came home that evening. I knew he had had a long and tiring day, occupied in important meetings. But his sad face told me his awareness about the day's calamity. We hugged each other in silence. I mentioned our new Pakistani friend at the gas station. He quietly got the car keys, reading my mind, and we both dashed out of the door.

"Come, come, how are you, my sister?" his gentle words came through our open car window. "What has happened to *Insan*-to humanity? What a disaster!" he emoted. I whispered to him, "Dear *bhai jan*- brother, don't wear your country's clothes, the *turban*, the long *zabba* and *patloon* right now. People won't understand. They are all confused and mad with vengeance. I want you to go away for few days, stay home maybe. I want you to be safe. OK?" His eyes welled. He nodded without any words, assuring me that he understood and would obey my request.

Aai's most precious advice kept repeating in my mind, "*In the 21st century, individual religion is not that important, the only religion that matters is of universal humanity.*" We drove home in silence. Finally a part of my lost peace of mind was found.

As soon as we returned home, I started writing a letter to assure Aai that we were all safe... Dear Aai, Namaskar[19] with all my love.

***

---

[19]Namaskar is a respectful greeting, a salutation in Hindu traditions.

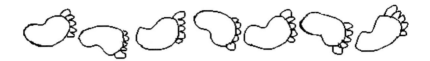

2002

Swati graduated from Cornell University with her Ph.D., another feather in her cap. We were so proud of her and happy that she was coming home at last after seven long years of hard work. We were thrilled that both daughters were nearby, Chitra working in Boston and Swati doing her post-doc at the University of MA in Worcester. They were both progressing successfully in their individual lives, and we were well-established in Nashua by then. I started teaching again as a pre-Kindergarten teacher. I also had joined a local artist guild and had my 2nd solo exhibition. Madhukar renovated our basement in order for me to teach Yoga at home. Without advertisement, my class was always full. Life was in full swing, Madhukar and I both loved our jobs, and daydreamed about retirement there in our new home 'Wind Song'. Chitra was engaged to Mark by then and would be married soon. Madhukar came home one day with the sudden news that his small company that was created by former Digital employees was being swallowed by Texas Instruments in Dallas.

***

We sat and discussed the pros and cons of uprooting ourselves once again. After enduring 36 years of harsh winters, the warmth of golden rays was very alluring. Madhukar had "retired" twice already, but he still was not ready to completely stop. He always thrived in his work, so we decided to take this challenge. He was to start the new job right away. We flew to Dallas the following week to explore and find a new home. "Jyoti, you look for the house, after all you are the one who really lives in the house; I only sleep there," his usual brainy solution to gently impose the task on me.

'How am I going to fulfill this difficult mission in just one week?' The thought already started worrying me as our plane landed in the Dallas airport. Madhukar's boss was living in McKinney, Texas, and had booked a hotel for us there. He had suggested a real estate agent in McKinney, so we decided to consult her. Amusingly, just like Nashua had been, McKinney had also recently been chosen as "the best town to live in."

I started exploring that same afternoon, looking at prospective houses. After three days, I narrowed the search to two homes, and Madhukar came with me to finalize the choice and then we made an offer. We did not hear from the seller right away, and I was getting restless. Time was running short. There was a lake near our hotel, so I decided to go for a walk. The overcast sky competed with my gloomy thoughts about the looming separation from my darling daughters and all the friends we would leave behind. The last time I had taken a walk was in Nashua, at the river near our house. The great blue heron had signaled me to stay put with his fixed one-footed pose. I was sure I would never see him again. The flat land of Texas dominated by the tumble weeds would be so far away, 2,100 miles away from the beautiful fauna and flora of New England! All the stories that I heard about 'rednecks' and poisonous snakes were scary enough!

I longed to see the pines, maples, and lilacs. Maybe we made a mistake! We should go back; we must go back! I should have gotten used to moving by now. In 37 years of marriage I had moved to so many homes. Dadar, Dombivali, Decatur, Framingham, Nashua ... I prayed to the Goddess to give me a signal that this was the right move. The quiet ripples of the water suppressed my turmoil and brought a calmness to me. Even though all the folks strolling around the lake greeted me with smiles and hellos, a habit that was rare with New Englanders, I wanted to see a familiar face. All of a sudden out of the corner of my eyes, came the familiar sound of wings, a symphony to my ears. A great blue heron landed gracefully nearby. He stretched his long neck as if questioning whether I recognized him. The big red spot under his sharp eyes mirrored the red Tilak on my forehead. My friend the great Blue Heron had come to me from so far away. I came to a standstill. My mind was singing with joy. Somewhere in the background Saint *Kabir* was laughing, '*Where are you looking for me, you idiot? I am right next to you. I am within you!*'

A big tidal wave of happiness drenched me. Mute dialogue with the blue heron began. No need for spoken words between us. He came here all the way for me. I melted in his beautiful blue shade. Without my knowledge my palms gather to pray. I was sure now that the decision to move was the right one. There is no moving, *the whole universe is my home*. A great blue messiah came all the way to remind me that. "*Sat Chidananda*"- everlasting pure joy is within you. I hear my Dada's kind voice as if he is standing near me. His forehead is adorned with the same red *Tilak* as mine. My quest is over. *I feel at home, home is where the heart is.*

"What in the world is this creature?" Startled by these words, I looked toward the voice. A man was standing behind me. His long white beard flowed gently, and a web of wrinkles covered his face. There was a twinkle in his eyes. This is how I first met Tom. He is astonished, "I have been coming to this lake for the last 25 years, but I have never seen this strange bird."

"That is because this angel arrived here for me." I told him the saga of our big move and why the great Blue Heron was here. He understood me right away and said, "I believe you because I have experienced similar phenomena in the past."

This is how I found a friend in our new town. That lake sure held some magic. Our offer on the house was accepted on the same evening. I knew that it was more than just coincidence. Next day we signed the papers, and the house was ours. Madhukar stayed in McKinney and I headed back to Nashua for the demanding preparation needed to sell Wind Song and get ready for Chitra's wedding.

The Wind Song house always full of gentle breeze. Every *vastu*, *a*bode, that we lived in had given us a unique gift. Our Decatur apartment gave me a *Maher*-mother's home of my lifelong friends Helen and Dean. Swati my first shining star- a jewel appeared in my world. Michael Road gave us many blessings: the kind friendship of neighbors Linda and David Doran, Chitra's birth; Madhukar's textbook on management science, he became the first president of our Marathi Mandal by election. Many famous dignitaries and scholars visited our Michael Road home. My favorites were the poet Shanta Shelke, actor Shrikant Moghe, and industrialist Abasaheb Garware. That tradition continued in Montgomery Road's *Whispering Oaks.* There we were visited by the writer *Goni* Dandekar, historian and writer Shahir Babasaheb Purandare, Swamini Pavitraji, Swami Partha Sarthi, and actress and singer Suhasini Mulgaokar. My Yoga studies and class started in full swing at the same house. Madhukar's successful career, and my being chosen as a contributor to the children's arts and crafts book, all occurred in Whispering Oaks.

Now the Wind Song house soon would be full of *Shehnai* melodies, the cherry on top of the sundae being Chitra's wedding to Mark in April 2002.

"Aai, Chitra got engaged..." I was on a long-distant phone call with my mother.

"Very nice, good news! Who is the lucky guy?" I could hear the joy in her cheerful tone. I knew my Aai would be truly supportive for this marriage, yet still I hesitated to reply. How was I going to tell my patriotic mother? She who had given up tea to protest the tax on tea, during the struggle against the British *Raj*! She would not even eat bread, which symbolized British Christian culture. The freedom fighters *Swatantyaveer Sawarkar* and *Lokamanya Tilak* had been her role models.

I took a deep breath and blurted out, "Our son in law Mark is *gora sahib* from England."
"Jyoti, in the 21st century, it's more important to cultivate *Vaishwik Manavatecha dharma,* the religion of universal humanity, rather than an individual religion," her firm words gave me all the assurance I needed. This was my mother, full of wisdom, and born way ahead of her time. When I told her that Swati did not want to get married, that time also, she had comforted me with her true belief, "Jyoti, not everybody is born to get married. Each person has her own life to lead according to their own core." She truly practiced Geeta philosophy in her everyday life. I was so grateful that she was my Aai.

Chitra gave me full freedom to design the whole wedding. She wanted me to create her wedding invitations, so I started thinking of drawing a bride doing *Gourihar pujan*, the intimate prayer done just before the wedding ceremony. The bride worships *Lord Shankara* and asks for a long life for her groom. I asked my older brother Anna to find out any more details about this tradition. So he went to a teacher's home who taught at *Veda Bhavan,* a famous institute in Pune where ancient Hindu scriptures are studied.

"Who is the son-in-law?" the teacher asked. Anna started telling him about Mark, that he was from England. Abruptly the teacher cut Anna off and told him that he would not give any information. The teacher gathered his hat and put on his shoes and stormed out. The Hindu religion is known for accepting other religions, and Anna was shocked to see this educated man react in such an orthodox manner. Anna quietly stepped over the threshold to return home, when he was stopped by the gentle voice of an elderly woman. The professor's mother gestured to Anna to come inside again. She then explained the importance of *Gourihar pujan* to him.

In India, a woman could become a prime minister! On the other hand it is indeed a sad misfortune that so-called illiterate women, but so intellectual and full of wisdom of my mother's generation went unnoticed by society.

***

Madhukar had been officiating Hindu wedding ceremonies for many years and had been very disappointed to have missed Tanuja's wedding. So he was thrilled now for Chitra's loving wish for him to officiate her marriage to Mark. Now the priest and the wedding planner were fully committed for the upcoming event. Madhukar would stay in Texas until a few days before the wedding; I was the one-woman band preparing the house for sale and get ready for wedding. I had volunteered as a chairperson for the Brihan Maharashtra convention in Boston a few years back; my responsibility was to create ambiance in the Hyne's Convention Center. That experience came in handy for me, giving me some unique ideas for the wedding hall. I threw myself entirely into this project. I had inherited both Dada's perfectionism and Aai's management skills, so I was well organized two days before the wedding. I was excited and eagerly awaiting the big day.

***

I was in the kitchen doing last-minute chores before the guests would arrive following day. I suddenly felt a loving hug from behind, Chitra must have quietly tiptoed into the house. It was the same loving hug she used to wrap around me when she got home from school. I wish I could keep her now in my arms forever. So many things I wanted to tell her, all the motherly advice. The thought that from now on she would be somebody's wife and not just my daughter was unbearable. Chitra had taken two days off before the wedding - a rare bonus for me. She was always so busy, traveling constantly for work, with no time at all for herself.

I wiped my tears before she could see and turned around, "Come on, we have to do *Mehndi*." I held Chitra's soft palm in my hand and began to draw a decorative design with henna. Her left foot began to move in a gentle rhythm that pulled me all the way back to Chitra's infancy, the same pulse of her tiny foot while I was nursing her. The same peace in the house, the universe filled with just my baby Chitra and me. I noticed that Chitra was unusually quiet today. Was she nervous?

'Babul Mora Naihar Chhooto Jaye'... My mind sped faster than a rocket to that wintery cold midnight in 1972, *Makar Sankranti.*

My contractions had started in full force. While next door Aunt Mari had offered wholeheartedly to keep Swati overnight, we decided that Madhukar would stay with Swati and I would go alone to the hospital. So again Madhukar could not be with me as I gave birth to our 2nd baby. Back when Swati was born, the hospital did not allow the father to be present in the birthing room.
I was all alone on the hospital bed, agitated, contractions rising every minute with unbearable pain. WCRB radio was playing classical music which soothed me a bit. Even though I was eagerly awaiting the new arrival, I was not sure if I could love this new baby as much

as I loved Swati. The birth went smoothly, and the doctor soon put my newborn baby on my stomach. Looking at this tiny bundle of God's miracle, my motherly love started overflowing like 'Old Faithful' again. I hugged my baby tight to my heart. The calendar on the wall flapped, showing Friday, January 14, and the clock struck one beat, announcing 2:30 a.m. I was delighted to have another baby girl. These two Devi's Avatars arrived on a Tuesday and a Friday; both days were dedicated for Goddesses. Madhukar had chosen a name already as Chitra, another constellation in the sky - Spica, as Swati was also named for the nearby constellation Arcturus. These two constellations are considered as sisters. Newborn Chitra's big round eyes shining brightly wiped away all my loneliness instantly. I felt bigger than the sky, Chitra making my universe complete. All my doubts were washed away when she latched onto my nipple and the milk started flowing like the river Ganga. Later that morning Madhukar came with Swati *tai*-a big sister. I could see from all the joy spilling from his face that he was also thrilled to have another daughter. The words flew out of his mouth euphorically, "Do you know that my mother is here?"

I was puzzled by his words, as my mother-in-law had died of a sudden illness four years ago. She was so very fond of girls, since she had two sons. I got a sweet taste of that fondness when I married into the Joshi family. She was delighted to hear about her first granddaughter's birth. Unfortunately, soon after that, without seeing Swati she left this world.

"My Aai came yesterday to our house. I asked her how she came and who sent her the plane ticket. She answered smilingly, 'Did you forget? I don't need a ticket now. I am going to stay with you permanently," Madhukar described his dream to me.

Since Chitra was born on the same day as his dream, Madhukar strongly believed that his mother had returned to us as Chitra. Later that summer his Aimee Aaji came from India to visit us. When she saw Chitra, she exclaimed, "Oh my, Madhu, she looks just like your Aai, she has the same smile!"

As soon as we came home from the hospital, I tossed away Dr. Spock's guide. I was quite confident about how to take care of my baby. Chitra was growing fast like a weed, strong and healthy.

"Aai, I am so happy that you took the responsibility of being my wedding planner. I love all the unique ideas you have." Chitra's words woke me up from daydreaming, making me aware that my baby had come a long way. The little girl had grown into a beautiful young woman, a well-respected manager in her company.

All the guests from out of town arrived in time to celebrate *Kelwan*, the traditional pre-wedding feast for the bride. There was no facility to cater typical Marathi specialties, so I happily I took over the task. *Gulabjam, shreekhand, gajar halwa, ras malai, and Burphi*, all the *Pancha Pakwans* a traditional feast of five deserts-along with Chitra's favorite dishes. My cousin sister Ushatai brought homemade puran poli, roti stuffed with sweet *basen* paste, all the way from Chicago.

April 28, 2002

We celebrated Mark and Chitra's wedding in full blast. I was grateful for all the help that my friends offered; I could not have done it alone. It made me sad that this would be the last time I would see all my friends for a while. Wind Song was sold just before the wedding. Madhukar left for Texas two days after Chitra's wedding, and I stayed behind to wrap up the last-minute things. I could not help but linger in the past 35 years of memories in beautiful New England.

Just yesterday I was a little girl playing with dolls. I had set up the doll house and broke it the very next minute without even thinking. Today that doll was old and tired. I was trying to get rid of all the stuff I had collected in my greed.

My hands shook while giving the items away one by one to Goodwill. My mind was silently chanting, *'idam na mama*[20] *, idam namama-It's not mine, it does not belong to me…*

---

[20] *Idam Na Mama* is a famous mantra recited at offerings to Agni the fire god. "O God! Whatever I have, really belongs to you, and I offer it all to you."

The mover's truck was in the driveway. Men started taking furniture out of the house. The house was empty in a matter of hours. That night I slept on a borrowed mattress from my neighbor Swarupa. Wind Song became a stranger. I felt like a trespasser, that empty abode shrilly echoing with only my own voice. For the first time in my adult life all the so-called necessities were not available to me. No phone connection, no TV, no fridge, no car, no keys. A momentary foretaste of detachment for *Vanprastha*[21].

***

Suhana safar...Mery Duniyaa, mere sapane, milege shaayad yahi - Perhaps I might find my world, my dreams here, on this beautiful journey. - A song from the Hindi movie, Madhumati

Tuesday, May 4, 2002

I started my weekly letter.

Dear Aai,

Namaskar with all my joy, love, and Peace.
Vasudhaiv Kutumbakam-The whole world is my family-repeating this famous mantra, I left Boston today, 4 hours of flying, 2000 miles away to McKinney Texas. My dear friend Dee came all the way from

---

[21] Vanaprastha - The stage of partial retirement from worldly life; vanaprastha is the third of four ashrams or stages of life in Hindu philosophy.

Framingham to take me to Boston. So I am writing you this letter from the airplane.

All my friends and my darling daughters are left behind. It feels like instead of Chitra, I am the one who is going to *Sasari*, my in-laws house. Times like this I don't know how you and Dada sent me so far away. You never once showed me the sorrow of our separation. How did you do it? Please give me your blessings so I can do the same with Swati and Chitra.

The next day after my wedding somebody asked my name and I blurted out, "Jyoti Deodhar!" the name that had been engraved on me from birth. I could not even utter my new identity of Shubhangi Joshi. The same thing happened today at the airport. My pen could not write the new address of our McKinney home. *8 Heathrow Drive, Nashua, NH* was branded in my mind. The beautiful wildflowers on the backyard hill that Madhukar cultivated so tenderly would always keep blooming in my heart.

Remember once, I had asked you, "It must have been very difficult when you and Dada set up your tent in Pune all over again after 50 years of living in Dadar." Your answer came so easily, "*Jyoti, this Parimal house in Pune is our very first home. We were always busy taking care for others, now I will have complete freedom in this home to be on my own.*" Aai, I saw your enthusiasm for new beginnings. Dada and you created your own *Vishwa* again in Pune. You are and will be always my mentors.

***

Once again, I started writing my diary regularly and it became my own friend. The days had moved in slow motion, yet it was almost a year already since we moved to McKinney. We knew it was not that easy to move at age 55+ to somewhere you don't know a soul. I tried to keep myself busy with gardening, listening to classical Indian music, painting, taking walks every day, and practicing yoga, etc. But it was not enough. Backache from my dislocated disc clung to me like a constant shadow. I had met lots of people but none of them were able to enter into the arena of friendship yet. I was getting depressed thinking of all the dear friends I left behind. In spite of Madhukar's belief that I can talk with anybody easily, even a sparrow or a crow, I am still kind of an introvert. I like my own quiet place. But sometimes the house gets too quiet. I was far from true friends. The whole day would pass without seeing a single person. I would be all alone at home. I was so desperate that I wanted to invite our mailman in for a cup of tea.

Remembering Kabir's Doha, *'Ghoonghat Ke Pat Khol Re Tohe'* - do away with your veil (illusion) and you shall meet your beloved (Divine)- I decided to stop moaning and find a solution. I remembered seeing a sign in the library about a local artist's club. The following morning, I went to join it and, on the way, stopped at the senior center in town to sign up as a volunteer. I enrolled in the community college for a graphic art course. I started enjoying my life as a student again in the college surroundings where I met wonderful professors and other art students. I finally found myself again.

Walking around the enchanted McKinney lake every morning became my passion. My darling daughters and dear friends from Boston were deeply rooted in my mind. My longing for them would melt away in the ripples, giving me soothing healing. I met lots of wonderful people on my walks. I used to see a woman with a big smile on her face. One day as we passed each other she said to me, "Now that I have seen you, I know my day is going to be perfect." I told her the feeling was mutual. I found out she was an art teacher. I met Britina last month, who asked me if I was a yoga teacher. My hand went to check on my forehead if by mistake I put a yellow sticky note announcing about my yoga class. She immediately joined my yoga class. The same thing happened with Tony, a piano teacher, and her husband, an artist, who were regulars on the lake. They not only became my students but also very close friends. Without any advertising my yoga class was full again. This lake had also given me a very special angel named Ann. A few months ago I spotted Ann. Her tall figure on the other side of the lake was easily visible. Our paths had crossed often. That day when she came closer, she stopped, and we chatted. Before I knew it, we became buddies. After reading *Autobiography of a Yogi* by Paramhansa Yogananda, she became fascinated with Indian philosophy. She stopped practicing

Catholicism and going to church. I used to look forward to our discussions on philosophy while walking and later meditating together under the tree on the bank of the lake. I was convinced that we moved to McKinney so that I could meet all the wonderful people at this lake.

***

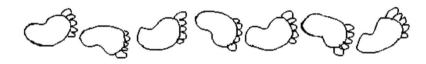

January 10, 2003

I woke up with a jolt. My flight was leaving in 8 hours. I was on my way to see Aai in India. I was feeling a little unsure of the trip. This was not the first time I was leaving Madhukar. He had always been very supportive of these trips for the last 19 years, so why was I restless now? Maybe because our anniversary was around the corner. We were still far away from our daughters. My mind was bothered by the thought of leaving my beloved behind to go to such a faraway place, out of nowhere words started dancing…

'While moaning and grumbling you turn off the alarm, even though far away I would be still locked in your embrace.

You would read the New Yorker in the bathroom,
While I would pound on the door,
Tossing your clothes everywhere, forgetting I would be watching you.

Throwing your wet towel on the bed after the shower...the mercury of my anger would rise so high that in a flash it would dry all its dampness.

Listening to Beethoven in the car,
I would be swaying gently in rhythm with you in the passenger's seat
When you returned from the office, tired and fatigued.
I would sit next to you, my eyelids fanning a gentle kiss of a butterfly.

Don't forget to light a candle at the dinner table, this Jyoti would be glowing only for you, only for you.

Think of me, remember me, when the jaswandi blooms, its red color seeping down into my veins.

When the birds come to the birdfeeder, my memory would perch on your shoulder.

When you would observe Venus on the horizon, I would be gazing at the same Venus.

I see you having a chuckle, for sending me far away, enjoying your freedom...
be aware I have locked you in the cage of my love, throwing the key away on the path of our seven lives together.

Maybe because of our long separations, whenever I was away in India, Madhukar would always write me love letters. My dear husband, a man of few words! Those letters became my treasure, more precious than all the jewels he showered on me. I had kept them all carefully in a walnut wooden chest he had bought for me in Kashmir. The carving was beautiful but no way near in comparison to his love, which carved itself as deep into my heart after reading the letters over and over.

His Marathi was eloquent and poetic. His professor *Shree Pu. Bhagavat* had wanted him to do his masters in Marathi. But at that time Madhukar's financial condition was very dire, and he asked Mr. Bhagavat, "If I major in Marathi, how would I earn my living?" During my more recent trips, however, he stopped writing because now overseas phone calls were much cheaper.

There would always be some kind of surprise gift waiting when I returned home. This time as soon as I entered the house, Madhukar stuffed a paper in my hand. I blossomed with joy reading his note. It was no ordinary note, but a true confession of missing me, solid evidence written in his beautiful handwriting. No wonder he called me almost every day. Pushing the jetlag away, that same night I scribbled something as if Madhukar were writing it himself in his diary:

A Wife Named Teacher

'Man is a student all his life' - Lokmanya Tilak's quote resonated in my ears. I didn't comprehend its full meaning until the very first day Jyoti became my wife. "Raja, I am telling you constantly, still you don't understand! Now listen to me." From that day on my coaching sessions started.

In the morning most people wake up to an alarm. But we don't have such an easy solution. Jyoti gets an urge to listen to Veda mantras before sunrise. The loud chanting pierces my sweet slumber at early dawn. I have bought her headphones, but she insists that the mantras should vibrate in our walls for *urja* (energy). She thinks it's her moral responsibility to wake up the whole house with spiritual music. She is very particular to listen to specific mantras each day. Monday is for Mahadev, Tuesday for Shree Sukta, Wednesday for Ganapati, Thursday for Vishnu Sahastranam, Friday for Devi, and Saturday for Hanuman chalisa. Even Sunday, my only day to sleep late, is not spared; I have to wake up to 101 chants of the Gayatri Mantra.

Frustrated, I walk into the kitchen to make chai. I see Jyoti meditating on a corner chair at the dining table. She likes her tea boiling hot and spiced with fresh ginger. So I put the kettle on and start pounding the ginger root. Her dhyan is disrupted and she makes her eyes even bigger. Her arms start signaling ferociously in the air, suggesting something to me which I am unable to hear over the harsh whistling of the kettle starts. I hurry to turn off the CD, and our day starts with the loud sirens of a cold war. I escape from the battlefield and run to the bathroom. I turn the shower on and start singing. When I was growing up, there was only a limited time to collect and store water from the city supply line, and only a bucket full of hot water was provided by my mother's coal stove.

"Mr. Joshi, Al Gore has warned us to conserve water! Besides, breakfast is ready so get dressed quickly," Jyoti yells.
She always insists that we eat breakfast together on Sundays. So like an obedient child I rush to the bedroom and start putting on my favorite red plaid shirt, brown pants, and whatever socks I can find. Pleased with my efficiency, I entered the kitchen like a hero.

"You still have no clue of matching clothes," Jyoti throws one glance at me. Before I got married, my closet held only a few choices. My shirts would be either white or off-white and the slacks would be black or gray. I am paying the price now of marrying an artist.

As I begin to eat, she inquires if I did Dhyan. I joke meekly, winking at her, "Dear, all my life I have been trying very hard to meditate on this Jagdamba (a fierce Devi who destroys demons) but no such luck." Jyoti ignores my playfulness and instead quizzes me, "Ok, listen to the Bhajan and at least tell me what raag[22] it is?"

"I only know one *Anurag-* referring to the faux anger of a lover's squabble," ... I gently throw a flying kiss at her.

"Come on, there is a furniture sale, we have to go. Our sofa is really old, and I noticed that Lila has exactly the same model as us." This is another of Jyoti insistences, not to have the same décor as others. So our house often is full of antiques from garage sales, things that people have gotten rid of.

You never know where she will see art, sometimes even in rags and trash. She does not throw anything away. One day after we ate pistachios, those shells appeared in our front yard in the form of

---

[22] Raag- In Indian classical music, a *rāag* consists of at least five notes, and each *rāag* provides the musician with a musical framework within which to improvise. Raags are played during a certain time of the day.

beautiful design. She is crazy about rocks and pebbles. Whenever we are traveling, I became a donkey, always carrying rocks and driftwood as souvenirs. After we come home, she washes and meditates on them. Revelation takes place and with few brush strokes or lines of her pen, they come alive into the form of an animal, or body parts. Our house is full of Feng Shui with dry twigs, pinecones, and stag horns. Normal people decorate the dining table with flowers; in our house you will find ginger roots, a shiny purple eggplant, or a red cabbage arrangement, under the guise of 'art'.

I never know when she will suddenly command me to stop the car, spotting a bird, flower, or a star. The other day she yelled while I was driving, "Oh, there is a full moon!"

"Where?? Where is it?" I jammed on the brakes, terrified that I had run over it.

"What do you mean where? Where else the moon would be, Dear? It's up there in the sky. I forgot that it's *Purnima* today. Give me your phone, I have to call the girls." She has created a moon club with other lunatics and has enrolled our daughters in it.

Every anniversary Jyoti gives birth to a new poem, to which I, of course, am the captive audience. I never know when she will get inspired by her muse. One time she bought fresh ears of corn for dinner, and as she took them out from her grocery bag she exclaimed, "I must paint a still-life of these beautiful yellow pearls. I don't belong to anybody right now, leave me alone until I am finished painting."

I am so brainwashed by her teachings that I am very restless when she is far away in Pune. I am not actually enjoying this vacation the way I had anticipated I would. I can't even throw my wet towel on the bed. It's not fun anymore without her scolding. I had gone to somebody's house for dinner the other day, and their blank white walls started closing in on me. Every differently colorful wall in our home that she begged me to paint way before it was in style, lured me back. But on my return, I was terrified by the silent house; there was no classical melody playing. I was truly missing her loving persona. I wanted her to come back right away!

***

March 2004

We were roaming in the Dallas arboretum when the cell phone rang. I knew it must be one of my girls calling. Chitra's voice clear and glowing with excitement, "You are going to be Aaji and Ajoba!" Madhukar's eyes welled up with tears. He could not talk. Madhukar's joy mirrored through my eyes. Delightedly we both hugged each other. I was so pleased to see my husband, a man of composure, become so emotional. This was happening more often nowadays. Last week when we were watching Elizabeth Taylor and Spencer Tracy's old movie 'Father of the Bride', the same thing happened; he teared up. I liked this new change. "*Finally you have become a real man!*" My hug became tighter around him.

Later we went to browse in the Arboretum's gift shop. I spotted a beautiful white angel sitting on a rock, holding a dove in her hand. I had stopped buying these kinds of knickknacks lately, but that angel kept luring me. I thought there was some connection between that guardian angel and today's good news. I carried her gently as we headed home. I found a perfect spot on my windowsill; the day was complete with her blessings. From then on, I became obsessed with angels. I would find them hidden in the form of twigs or rocks and bring them home to make them visible to others with my brush strokes.

Chitra's good news gave birth to my muse again. I started painting only one subject, 'Mother and child'. One early morning a heartfelt image appeared in my mind. It was not a daydream. I shrugged my shoulders and started setting the breakfast table on the deck, but that image kept flashing, and would not allow me to eat. I rushed in the kitchen and jotted that intuition on a note, sealed it in an envelope and kept it in my shrine, in front of Devi. The next six months seemed like six years. I found every excuse to visit Chitra for pampering. I planned a full shebang of a *dohalejevan*, baby shower. My dear friend Manda, whom I met long before Chitra was even born, happily offered her house in Sudbury, Massachusetts. She was my very first Maharashtrian friend in Framingham, we were living in apartment, a short transition until we could move in our new house. The bell rang and two Indian ladies waited at the threshold of my apartment. This was a rare occasion for me, since there had been no Indians in Decatur, Illinois. I could not get over the excitement when I heard them welcoming me in Marathi. Over the ensuing decades our friendship blossomed deeply. My girls called her Manda Maushi. She full heartedly agreed to offer her beautiful home for the celebration. Finally, September came. My plane landed in Boston a few days before Chitra's due date.

***

September 21, 2004

I tried to push the morning faster along. "I am too excited to drive." I handed the car keys to Swati and we were on our way to Beth Israel Hospital in Boston. My phone rang as she parked the car in the Longwood Ave garage. Mark was on the phone, "It's a boy!!"

Swati and I literally jumped up and down in the parking lot. Little baby feet would be trotting soon in our home after 33 years! I took the envelope from my pocket that I had carried so carefully from Texas. *A sweet secret, when I saw a little baby boy, with a lock of thick black hair.* I gestured to Swati to read my note and said, "Let's hurry inside first. I will explain it to you all together."

'Kal pahile mi Swapna, gade - I saw a beautiful dream yesterday', Song sung by Asha Bhosale, resonated in my mind... Tears of joy flowing, I saw a little baby, my Bal Krishna.

***

December 1970, Bombay Airport

We had just arrived for Madhukar's younger brother Vijay's wedding. Swati was a little over a year old. As soon as she saw my Aai, she dove into her arms as if she'd known her always. My mother, who was usually calm and composed, burst into joy of tears, and showered her with kisses. Then she told me, "Jyoti, I had a dream just before Swati was born. I was holding Swati on my lap and we were sitting under a Prajakta tree. The heavenly flowers started showering gently on us."

Aai's words kept ringing in my ears as Swati and I approached the delivery room. Chitra's doctor was still doing her last-minute care after the birth, so we were not allowed to see the newborn baby and mother yet. I picked up an old magazine in the waiting room but could not concentrate on reading.

"*Maza chakula, maza sona, maza gundyabhau* (my munchkin, my gold nugget, my sweet bundle of joy)!" a cascade of adoring Marathi words gently rocked my ears.

After Chitra was on her own, Marathi vanished from her vocabulary. But today that long hidden mother tongue erupted from her lips.

All the intense hospital odors dispersed instantly. Long live *Matrubhasha*, (Mother Tongue). Little Jeevan's *avatar* filled the house with a blissful *Chaitanya*, exuberance. While giving him an herbal oil massage, his baby cooing brought me joy.

"Oh *babuly* is awake, his diaper needs to be changed, my little precious prince must be hungry, don't cry my honey." My constant monologues.

Jeevan had rekindled the dormant *vatsalya*, motherly love in my heart. I was feeding Chitra almond kheer, dinkache laddus and other typical Indian dishes to aid in her new role as a nursing mother. Ajoba could not wait any longer in Texas. I was happy to see Madhukar rushed back to Boston a lot earlier than planned. I was admiring how he was handling the newborn. Jeevan's tender head resting on his shoulder, he started *Shatapawali*[23]. But I felt a little uneasy watching his fast pacing, something was bothering him. I rescued sleepy Jeevan to his bassinet. I went to the kitchen to do the dishes. Madhukar followed me there and turned me around lacing his fingers in my wet hands.

---

[23]Shatapawali is a Marathi term which refers to an age-long Indian custom of taking a stroll after a meal. The word literally means "walking 100 steps."

He made me sit down. "Jyoti, your Aai had a stroke, she is in the hospital in Pune. Your brother-Aba called last week. He was concerned about Chitra so warned us not to tell you and Chitra then. We decided that I should tell you this in person rather than over the phone. But now Aai is very serious and she is counting her last breaths. I know you would want to be with her. So I hurried here. I brought your passport and booked an airline ticket for you." He poured all that in one breath.

I was numb to hear about Aai's condition. I had promised Aba, after Dada's death that no matter what, I would be there by Aai's side when she is at her last moments. I froze with fear that she would be gone just as Dada had done. It tore me apart that I would leave Chitru and baby Jeevan so soon. I had planned to stay with Chitra until she felt comfortable handling the baby on her own. I remembered how nervous I was when Swati was born with nobody to guide me. Madhukar had to go back to Texas. Seeing my turmoil of next few days, Chitra assured that she would be fine and told me in no uncertain terms to go to my Aai. Mark was going to take some days off. Swati was also ready to help.

***

October 13, 2004

My morning had been busy in making lots of food for Chitra to freeze. There was no time to think of anything else. Suddenly I realized it was my birthday today! All those years had passed by, I had become a grandmother, but I still turned into a little girl on my birthday.

I always called my Aai for her blessings on my birthday and thanked her for bringing me into this beautiful world. This time I couldn't call her personally or tell her that she had become a *Panjibai*, a great grandmother.

"Aai, I know you are torn between Aaji and Chitra. I want you to be with your Aai, so go without worrying about her. I will take care of my little sister." Swati's promise resonated in my ears. I woke up at early dawn, Jeevan a sleepy head next to me. I had brought him into my bed again last night so Chitra could have a few hours of sleep after his last feeding. I had started this routine since she came home from the hospital. I got so attached to this joy of bundle in my bed. Each morning would trumpet me with his cooing and greet me with his dark brown eyes.

I gently kissed his head, the touch of his silky hair softer than peacock feathers pulling me more into deep affection. How can I leave him? My heart ached. Apple of my eyes, his fussy crying, his playfulness while he was awake, his tight fist around my pinky, everything was so precious. His yawns would give me a taste of Yashoda's Vishwadarshan[24].

His tiny aura had captured my heart. The slow rhythm of Jeevan's soft breathing felt like a soothing breeze before the storm that I was going to face soon. I panicked. My mind got stuck in a whirlpool of anxiety and I went way back in time.

Thirty-seven years ago Madhukar and I are at the airport about to leave for America. My Aai embracing me in a bear hug, Dada's trembling hands patting me on the back, their teary eyes flooding my own eyes. How long would our separation last? Tomorrow when Jeevan wakes up, I would be thousand miles away from him. When I see him again, he won't even recognize me. *This wheel of life would go on churning. I was trying to catch the center point of that circle - my aging Aai. My Aai who was counting her last few breaths before making room for this newborn soul Jeevan.*

The thought of leaving Chit and her baby made me stumble on the doorstep as I was leaving for airport.

My plane was not going to take off for another 3 hours. My ears turned off to all the announcements in the airport… all I could hear was Aba's warning, "Aai is lingering on the threshold of death, Jyoti, so be prepared for the chance you might not get here in time to see her."

---

[24] Vishwadarshan- Krishna opened his mouth in front of his foster mother Yashoda, who sees the entire Universe inside him.

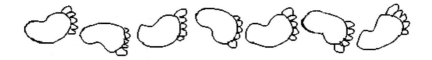

Harwale te gawasale ka? Lost has been found or is it what has been found is already lost?- songwriters P. Savalaram and Vasant Prabhu

October 19, 2004

I reached Bombay early dawn on the 15th of October. I took a bus with Aba from the airport directly to Pune, a three-hour drive. I rushed to her hospital right away. All the nurses welcomed me with relieved smiles, "Aaji has been waiting for her dear daughter." I don't know how long I sat there gratefully holding Aai's hand. But deep down I knew this wouldn't last long. How could a mere machine support somebody larger than the sky and taller than Mt. Everest?

My Aai who came first in the district at her middle school finals but had to leave the school after 7th grade, so her brothers could get a higher education. But she did not need those books to be a learned person. I had to go across seven seas to see all her qualities. It took me a long time to realize her love for me, hidden underneath her stern face. I thought I became an artist on my own. But she was the one from whom I inherited all my creativity. She was the one who taught me the real art of living. I am what I am today because she is my Aai, she was my guru and always will be.

Next morning, I woke up already depressed, because even in my sleep my mind was smoldering with the sadness. I started doing my morning chores like a robot. Thought I would go for a morning walk. I got ready, but I couldn't put one foot in front of the other, something was stopping me. In that moment of hesitancy, the phone rang.

The doctor was calling to let us know that Ai was in her last moments. I went numb. I said to Aba, "Let me go, since I'm ready. You do what needs to get done." I rushed out the door.

When I stepped in the hospital room, the medical staff told me that she had taken a turn for the worse and had slipped into a coma. They estimated she would only be alive for another few hours. I urged the clock on the wall to beat slower. The thought of losing her stabbed me with a deep loneliness. I had experienced the same isolation at Chitra's birth, all alone in the hospital room, painful contractions my only companion. But then I was anxiously waiting for new life to begin, and now I was anxiously dreading a life about to depart.

My dearest Aai would no longer be in my life, going far beyond where my weekly letters could reach her. There is so much I wanted to tell her. Four days ago when I arrived, I didn't talk too much because she needed her rest. All these 37 years so far away from her had taught me so much about her. I felt very helpless, didn't know how to cope. Then I remember what my brother Anna had told me, "When the last breath comes, pray to Dattatray, the God of tranquility." Unfortunately, I didn't know the correct mantra, so to keep my mind calm I gathered my courage and started to chant desperately, "Bhur bhuv swaha." The Gayatri Mantra always gave me strength.

Aai's breathing became extremely slow. Her chest was moving up and down when I entered her room this morning, but now it was still, and her throat started bobbing up in a very strange rhythm. Abruptly I became very calm. The fatal agony stopped. The future, the past, and the present melted in a serene tranquility. Somewhere in the unknown realm I began to float. *"Om Puurnnamadah Puurnnam Idam...the outer world and the inner world are completely full of Divine Consciousness."*

*"Asato Ma Sadgamaya Tamaso Maa Jyotir Gamaya.
Om shanti, shanti, shantihi."* ...*From falsehood lead me to truth, From darkness lead me to light. Om peace, peace, peace.*

With that Shanti Mantra my hand involuntarily ceased patting her forehead and at same time her breathing stopped. The last few days of sheer agony and torment disappeared; my mind was calm. I realized that I had not uttered these mantras lately. I was totally convinced that as she was passing from this world, Ai had made me chant to give me comfort. I knew she had found the freedom and peace of infinity.

On my return flight, as our plane took off, the words raced from my pen.

*You thought you had cut off my umbilical cord right at birth,
but it was only an illusion!
I look in the mirror only to find your reflection.
My evening shadow takes your shape.
My proud gourmet cooking merely gives my guests
the taste of your hands.
I am stumbling at every step to follow your advice.
I thought that I was a self-made liberated woman,
free to do whatever I desired.
But now that you have left this earth,
I realize the naked truth,
that I am still tangled in the umbilical cord.*

When I was back in McKinney, the bereavement was excruciating. Finally, I got fed up with myself, of my anguish. I was going to follow Aai's advice: don't sit idly, use your time to do something positive. I decided to fulfill the promise I gave her last time I had visited of publishing all of my letters to her over the years into a book. That's how '*Patzad*', my first book was born.

***

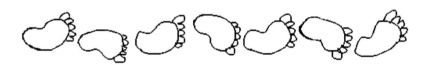

February 1, 2006

"Jyoti, now we are going back to Boston."

I was startled to hear Madhukar's cheerful announcement. The knot of the long five years in McKinney loosened easily. The sky was not enough to fill my joy. In fact this decision was taken before we moved to Texas. We knew that we were going to be back in Massachusetts someday. I remember that day vividly. I had told him firmly,

"Raja, when your job takes you anywhere in the world, I will tag along with you happily, but when you retire, I need to settle down near my darling daughters!"

All my American friends would get together on holidays with their families. They would always invite me, and I thoroughly enjoyed those celebrations, but I was still plagued by the thought that I didn't have blood relatives here in America. I was separated from my parents and did not want my daughters to be separated from us.

Hearing his decision of retirement my mind started swaying. Little Jeevan danced in front of me. My heart longed to take him in my embrace. I couldn't sleep a wink at night, "*I could have danced all night!*" I started daydreaming… I am giving him a bath, feeding him dahi bhath, his favorite meal of yogurt mixed with soft rice, telling him stories from the Ramayana and Mahabharata, pushing his stroller…I would be so happy in his company. I did not know when the sun peeped. I got ready and drove to the realtor Sharon's office.

"We want our house on the market," I declared.

"Jyoti, why in the world do you want to move back to Boston? You are retired, enjoy all the warm weather and sunshine. Why would you even think of leaving all those riches, not to mention you have a beautiful house here. Boston is an old ancient town."

"Sharon, my whole life is there," I calmly replied, explaining to her that Jeevan's name means 'life'. I could see from her expression that she did not agree with me. I knew the coming days would be busy with the chores of moving, but with the thought of this long-awaited migration I floated like a feather all the way home. This migration was the first in my life that was a wave of bliss.

The next day Chitra arrived with Jeevan as planned. It was Jeevan's first visit to Texas. I welcomed them by pouring some milk on her feet and doing *Aarti*, then I circled the coconut three times around them to keep one's evil eyes away before they entered the house. Jeevan stretched both his arms and leaned towards me. His adoring embrace woke up the overflowing grandmotherly affection in me. Even mere cinders are hot inside. I knew right away that his being close by would give me warmth in the harshest winter months in Boston. Sharon needed us to sign some forms for the sale and was on her way to the house. I couldn't wait to have her meet my prince charming. The bell rang.

Jeevan followed with his baby steps as I opened the door. Sharon was standing at the door. Jeevan greeted her with his million-dollar giggles and started his baby talk. Pink cheeks, big dark brown eyes, and pitch-dark hair. She was completely mesmerized by him. Spontaneously the words came out of her mouth,

"Jyoti, I truly understand why you want to go back to Boston. If this little fellow were my grandson, a thousand elephants would not be able to pull me away from him."

I nodded to her with glee, "I told you so!"

***

September 2016, McKinney

It was a hot Sunday morning. Ann, Madhukar and I were walking in the woods behind the lake. I knew that our walks together on this road were going to end soon. I was so grateful for Ann's friendship. I knew in our very first meeting that our rapport was definitely not a coincidence. That lake had a sublime *shakti* and I had met several wonderful people on its shores. But Ann was the only one whose face would be engraved in the mirror of my mind. After our first casual meeting, I went to the lake the next morning hoping to bump into her again. As I saw her approaching me, she spoke the language of my heart, "Jyoti, I too was hoping to bump into you today." Our conversations covered lots of avenues of theology and Indian philosophy. It is not often that one meets a traveler on the journey whose goal is the same. Her thoughtful advice would give me strength to establish myself in this new land. I had never followed any swamis, but secretly I started looking to Ann as my Guru. We would sit on the bank of lake to meditate. We never went to each other's house or attended any parties together. The lake became our friendship's abode. "Your Madhukar is a wise man," she always admired him.

The thought of our walks together ending plunged me into melancholy. Another separation. How many friends I had left behind? Childhood friends from Narayan Niwas, friends as a newlywed in Dombivili, friends in our first home in Decatur, and all those dear friends in Framingham, Nashua, and now McKinney. How many times I pitched the tent only to fold it.

"Ann, we are moving back to Boston," I confessed, followed by uncontrollable sobbing.

"Don't get sad my dear friend, you know our friendship was not just serendipity. I was extremely lucky to find a Guru like you Jyoti!" Her words startled me. I started laughing, "What are you talking about Ann? I was the one who considered you as my Guru!" We both giggled through our tears.

Soon the day of our return to Boston arrived, and she came to bid me goodbye. My eyes welled. When would I see her again? Waves of anxiety lapped me deeply. Without any words, I hugged her so tightly as if never to let go.

"Jyoti, please don't be sad. It was a divine plan that we met. Whether or not we meet again in this lifetime is not that important. The goal was achieved." Ann calmly unlocked herself from my hug. *Why did I not meet Ann earlier? I would have packed her valuable message in my sack and carried it with me every time I was on an exodus, and the separations from friends would have been a lot easier.*

***

Norton, November 15, 2006

Dawn caressed me as I opened the kitchen windows. My garden in the backyard was still sleepy. Suddenly under the lush green leaves, a little jasmine bud burst to greet me, with its intoxicating perfume. Later, as I was driving to the pool during a traffic jam, the window of the car in the next lane rolled down and two dimples burst into a giggle - my daughter Swati going to her nearby office! My universe was filled with joy.

Our first Diwali with family together in 5 years was just around the corner. I started making all the traditional sweets and spicy dishes, like laddus and karanjis, but my heart was already full of delight. I had felt since we came back, that Diwali was at my house every day, our darling daughters nearby, my favorite son-in-law as I always called him, and of course the apple of my eye, Jeevan.

***

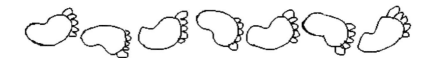

February 14, 2007

Madhukar was not keen on celebrating birthdays. Our birthdays were with a week of each other, but he would still forget mine. Yet somehow, he always remembered Valentine's Day. This morning was no different. We were still in bed when he whispered, "Don't make dinner tonight. Do you know what day today is?" "At last there is a little flicker at the end of the tunnel," I muttered back to him with giggles. Instead of breakfast, I scribbled a short note - a porridge of sweet words for him at the table.

'If you can unravel all 40 years of our entanglement,
You will only find one hidden magnet that has been pulling you.
From daybreak through the sleepy night it's been brushing at your feet like a cat.
When we take our evening stroll, our arms touch each other gently, like shadows.
You might have listened to my love song but ignored it,
Like the unheard ocean waves resonating in a conch.
Raja, it's my unconditional love that dances to the rhythm of your breath.

***

January 2008

"Jyoti, can you please verify the checkbook? Something is not right," Madhukar complained from upstairs in a tense tone.

"What's the matter with you? That's the same thing you said last month when the bank statement came. Maybe I should take it over like I used to," my annoyance was competing with the stamping of my footsteps on the stairs.

Lately he was behaving strangely. Just two days ago, I had to drive 30 miles to his office because he had lost his car keys. I told him to look everywhere, to no avail. When I got there, I checked in the jacket he was wearing and found it in the pocket.

We had always travelled whenever we could. Like the birds during Boston's wintery cold, we decided to migrate south to Miami for a few days. Our plane was delayed, and we didn't land until 11 p.m. Both of us were exhausted. We had left Norton very early in the morning. While Madhukar was adjusting his driver's seat in the rented car, I gave the command to our GPS to go to the hotel. He could not reverse the car and get out of the parking lot.

"What kind of car is this?" He became angry and started yelling at the car. I became alarmed by his shouting and cajoled, "Why don't I drive, and you navigate?" and took over the steering wheel. Finally, we reached our hotel. He fell asleep right away but the thought that he was unable to drive shoved my sleep away. Something else had happened just the week before on our way to the Natick Mall. We had lived in Framingham for 32 years and could have driven there with eyes closed. But that day he missed the exit and he got confused and didn't know how to get back to the mall. I told him to turn left at the signal, but he couldn't figure that out. "How can I turn the car there?"

His confused inquiry interrupted my peace of mind with lots of red signals. While going back to Norton another incident happened. Not only did he not stop for a pedestrian crossing the road, but he honked loudly at him. I was frightened by his action. What was wrong with him? Madhukar would always stop for people even when they were jaywalking. He also would always yield for drivers who wanted to make a left turn. He had an excellent driving record as did I, due to his teaching. Where did that Madhukar disappear to? What's wrong with him? I was caught in a net of unanswered doubts. "You should have let that person cross," I tried to make him understand, but he told me to be quiet, and to avoid more arguments I swallowed my retort. Then I saw a blue light spinning behind us. The police officer gave him a ticket for speeding and Madhukar continued his growls all the way home.

Now in Miami he was acting similarly. I was worried that something was not right. But the next morning there was no trace of any difficulty in his driving. He must have been tired, I tried to convince myself.

Our hotel was right on the ocean front and we would walk on the beach to our heart's content…

High tides chasing each other. Sea foam gently floating on the waves. Our sneakers' motifs on the wet sand. The sandpipers etching beautiful calligraphy with their tiny claws. White shells exposed by the receding tides, mica shimmering. Ballet of sea gull wings and the egret's graceful neck. The ocean's concerto was indeed a masterpiece. I was intoxicated with thirst for the sea. If I woke up in the middle of the night to use the bathroom, I would peek through the window to see the silver streak of the moon still riding on the waves. I kept staring at the ocean, mesmerized by its vastness, its constant beating at the sand bank. When would this infinite yearning end?

Eventually I noticed that this bliss of being with my soulmate near the ocean was shrinking. Whenever we were traveling by car, Madhukar was always eager to drive, and I was happy as a clam being chauffeured. But on this trip, his enthusiasm was vanishing. The sunny nature of his soul hid behind clouds of melancholy. His thundering laughter would spark into angry lightning.

I was deep into my thoughts standing in the veranda as the night spread its darkness. Our room was on the 13th floor, a number that has always been lucky for me since I was born on the 13th of October. The beach was doused in starlight. The waves turned into silvery molasses. Their primordial sound of Omkar echoed in the surroundings. Orion appeared in the sky and then out from the night's womb emerged the brightest star Vyadha. I don't know why but it seemed Vyadha was warning me of a storm ahead. That very moment I decided that as soon as we returned back home, I would take Madhukar to see a doctor.

***

September 2008

Ever since we had moved to Norton, I was urging Madhukar that instead of working, he should pursue his hobbies. He officially retired from Texas Instruments in 2006, which was his third retirement!

But his constant refrain was, "I must find a job!" Texas Instruments had a branch nearby us, and his old boss told him there was a job there waiting for him. Madhukar was thrilled, but when we returned back to Boston, he found out that the branch had recently closed. He felt betrayed. I tried to make him understand that his former boss probably didn't know about the current situation. His boss valued Madhukar's professional ability, and their relationship was good; he would not do such a thing. But Madhukar could not face reality and became very depressed. His dream to work continuously could not be fulfilled.

"I am going to work until the end, just like Professor Deming[25]!" He had excitedly announced when he got back from Deming's lecture in 1980. All evening he had talked about nothing but Mr. Deming, and from then on, he became Madhukar's mentor.

I assured him that he would find another job easily, like before. He was constantly worried that we won't have enough money to survive. On the contrary, Madhukar had invested brilliantly and there was no problem at all, but his unfounded worried obsession continued. His glass became half empty. Little things started to annoy him. His easy-going nature disappeared.

So one day I handed him a pen and paper and asked him to list all the assets in his life. He just sat there, rubbing his hands for a long time. I left the room. When I returned later, the paper was on the table full of remarks I hurriedly started reading...
1. I have a beautiful and loving wife named Jyoti.
2. Swati and Chitra, my daughters, are smart and successful in their careers.
3. My son-in-law is educated, intelligent and good hearted.
4. Jeevan my grandson is adorable.
5. We have a beautiful home to live in.
6. By god's grace, we have enough money in the bank.
7. We are surrounded by wonderful friends.

His note assured me that he was ok, just going through a difficult time. There soon followed a lucky opportunity. His old boss from Digital had formed a company and urged Madhukar to join, so he became a consultant at A123. The commute was long, but he didn't mind, and he worked only four days a week, giving us long weekends to enjoy ourselves. He was almost his old self again most of the time.

Then he had to go to China on a business trip. He had gone on many business trips over years, but for some reason I was extremely worried about his long trip. How would he manage on his own in an

---

[25] William Edwards Deming was an American engineer and statistician. He helped develop the sampling techniques still used by the U.S. Department of the Census and the Bureau of Labor Statistics.

unknown environment? In that stressful state of mind while I was out on an errand, I missed a step and fell down. I had broken my ankle and was confined to a wheelchair for the next 10 days. His flight was early dawn the next morning. He was hesitant to leave me in that condition, but I convinced him to go. I was touched by his concern. I was happy to see him return safely a week later and kept blaming myself for doubting him. He had loved China but did not get to do much sightseeing due to the very tight schedule, so he planned a trip for us for the following year, October 2009.

Just a week before we left for China, we had our appointment at the world-famous Framingham Heart Study. We were registered in the Omni heart study since we had lived in Framingham. Aside from the physical tests we had also undergone mental examinations for many years. This time we were going to see a neurologist, and when I entered his office, I found that the brain specialist was an Indian man, Dr. Nair. So I took advantage of the visit to express my concerns about Madhukar's spurts of moody and confused behavior. After listening to his symptoms, Dr. Nair had a suspicion of early dementia. I told him about our trip abroad. He immediately said, "If his behavior continues then bring him back here right away after you return, but Mrs. Joshi, let me warn you that airports are the worst places for these kinds of patients. The hubbub can make them more confused." I told him I would be on guard and take good care of him. I decided not to tell my girls until further evidence of this diagnosis.

***

After 18 long hours of air travel, we were exhausted, not to mention jet lag. It was our first dawn in Beijing. Madhukar woke up and went to the bathroom. but soon he returned back to bed. I was a sleepyhead and thought he was tired like me. But he started pacing back and forth.

"Jyoti, where is the toothpaste?" his question startled me awake. We had traveled all over the world together, and it was an unwritten rule that the toothpaste was always packed in the leather toilet kit.

I kind of ignored it and put the toothpaste on his brush and started singing an old Bollywood song, *'Jarurat hai, ek pativrataki, jo seva karegi patiki. I am in a desperate need of a wife who is devoted and would offer her services to her husband.'*

One thing that kept bothering me was that since we had started on the trip, he had been extremely quiet. He did not say one single "hi" or "hello" to our fellow travelers. Usually he would become the leader of the group with his talkative nature within the first 5 minutes. I choose to disregard it because I was experiencing the same fatigue from the long flight.

"Raja, I charged the battery all night. Can you please put it back into the camera?" I could see from the corner of my eye that he turned to pick up the camera. I collected other essentials for our day tour, hung the pocketbook on my shoulder, and made sure I had the room key. Shutting the door behind us, we stepped out toward the breakfast buffet.

There was a feast set in a very artistic way on the long table, laden with extraordinary Chinese cuisine which we were not accustomed to. 'Eat all you want' - I read the sign and decided to obey it. We did not like the Korean food on the flight, and I was ravenous. Madhukar was ahead of me in line. He stood frozen in front of the buffet. Finally he took a cup and poured muesli into it, ignoring the bowls. He moved further and started pouring passion fruit juice into a soup bowl instead of a glass. I could see he was totally baffled. I rushed to him,

"Dear, why don't you go find a table for us and I will bring your breakfast to you? I know what you like." I vividly remembered that on one of my trips to India, I was extremely confused for few days. Then I realized it was a side effect of the anti-malarial pills and I stopped them immediately. But on this trip that was not the case. Still in denial, I blamed Madhukar's behavior on jet lag and moved on.

Our bus reached Tiananmen Square, the Gate of Heavenly Peace. Our tour guide started telling us, "Tiananmen Square is the largest city square in the world, and it has been the site of several important events in Chinese history." I took out the camera to take pictures, but alas, there was no battery in it. Suddenly I remembered that he had been bending down looking for something in the hotel room that morning. So he had not put the battery in after all. The next few minutes were wasted in my fury at him. I tried to control myself and called the hotel desk to explain the situation and asked them to look for that tiny battery. Within an hour, the hotel's taxi service delivered the battery to me with a bill. I was annoyed that I had to pay such an expensive penalty but the at the same time I was quite impressed with Chinese efficiency.

"Airports are a major culprit in making these types of patients confused," Dr. Nair's words echoed in my head. My mind went wild with fear. From now on I would have to be extra cautious on this trip. I would have to take the lead and take good care of Madhukar, releasing him of any responsibilities. I noticed that he had a hard time in public restrooms, making our group late. He just could not handle it. I tried to cover up for him but later it became very difficult for me to find a new excuse every time we had to wait for him. At the hard climb at the Great Wall, I could only go to a few points because of my back problem. But amazingly, he climbed to the highest point that tourists were allowed, without any apparent difficulty. After a week, he got used to the tour's schedules and became much more like his old self. Still, I kept reminding myself, that I must make an appointment for him to see Dr. Nair as soon as we reached home. I started jotting down all of his behavior issues: lack of following simple instructions, confusion, no cognitive thinking, etc.

After returning from China I expressed my concerns to my daughters. "Aai, you know how daddy is absentminded always. You are worried for nothing," Swati and Chitra both tried to convince me. But deep in my gut I knew that this was beyond simple absentmindedness. I made appointment for Madhukar with Dr. Nair for my peace of mind and had no inkling of the avalanche that was about to bury me.

***

Breakfast was merely a habit that morning. She could not even taste her favorite hot ginger tea. She tried to calm herself with a flute and tabla melody, another favorite part of her morning rituals. But within a few moments a stream of tears started pouring through the melody. A tsunami of deep anxiety burst out.

'My beloved, please let me have your robust company all my life, please don't leave me. Let my suspicion be wrong. Devi give me strength. Please fill him with your shakti.'

The clock was ticking fast. She made sure they would be there on time for his appointment. Dr. Nair's office was in Quincy, about 30 miles away. He was dead set against seeing the doctor, but she convinced him in the end.

All his wisdom and shining intellect, where had it gone? He was still working in the office, so where was this confusion coming from? She discovered in the very first week of her marriage that her husband was an absent-minded professor. But his recent behavior was not just being forgetful; there was something seriously wrong. While he was grumbling in defiance, she kept urging him, "Raja, listen, we are just seeing the doctor in case. God forbid, if this is the indication of any unknown ailment, we could find a solution." In spite of all her assurances to him, she herself was not sure if she could face the dark shadows of the outcome of this visit.

***

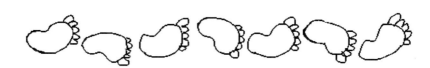

November 2009

Dr. Nair told Jyoti that the cognitive and physical assessments would take at least three hours, and he advised her to go out and treat herself for a cup of coffee at a nearby cafe. She called one of her friends who lived in Quincy, whom she had not seen in a long time. Her friend was concerned about why she would bring Madhukar such a long distant for checkup. Jyoti tried to explain but her jaw locked, and all the things she wanted to say started choking her. She could not utter the truth, could not confide in her friend. Feeling cornered, she gathered all her courage and begged her friend to keep this to herself and finally told her the reason for the visit to the clinic. She felt guilty while explaining, feeling uncomfortable as a mother would be talking of her misbehaving child.

She went back to the clinic. Madhukar was still being tested, including an MRI and cat scan of Madhukar's brain. Dr. Rosenthal, the chief psychiatrist asked him lot of questions, but it took him so long to answer that after 4 hours, a simple test of drawing a clock to show a particular time, was giving this gold medalist difficulty. Seeing that, Dr. Rosenthal kindly decided to relieve Madhukar from anxiety.

"It is definitely the beginning of Alzheimer's," Dr. Nair announced harshly, in a matter-of-fact tone! She and Madhukar had hardly entered his consulting room. His bluntness hammered her like a judge delivering a sentence. They did not have any time to sit down and digest his verdict. She wished he could have showed some compassion and shared his results with her alone at first. She would have gently passed on the diagnosis to her beloved. Madhukar became very furious when he heard Dr. Nair forbidding him to drive. He was given a prescription for Namenda pills, but nobody could prescribe any medicine for her sufferings.

Now he would be added to the sum of victims of Alzheimer's. A statistical survey would count Madhukar as only another digit. She did not know anybody close who was suffering from this disease. Her awareness was only from TV ads. She knew it would affect his memory but had no idea what else he would suffer. As they were leaving, she saw a book on the doctor's shelf, *The Everything Health Guide to Alzheimer's Disease*. She feebly asked the doctor if she could borrow it. As soon as he nodded, she snatched it on their way out as a trapped animal in a cage would see a hidden open door of escape. She didn't hesitate to complain to the secretary at the desk about his bedside manners.

She went to the elevator; Dr. Rosenthal was also waiting to go down. He smiled at her. "Mrs. Joshi, we will take care of your husband, but who is going to take care of you? Don't forget to look after yourself otherwise you as his caretaker will also became a victim," he warned her. She was baffled by his advice. *Take care of myself? Why do I need taking care of?*

***

"I don't have a job because I am not worthy. That's why I can't find a job." The obsession of those negative thoughts nagged at him when they moved to Boston. He became so paranoid. His rational thinking began to ebb. Was that the beginning of his Alzheimer's? She pushed away the swell of doubts in her mind. She was going to throw herself physically and mentally with all her ability into his care. She would not keep a single stone unturned. She knew her Devi would guide her to the remedy. She was going to be his boat and a bridge across his Alzheimer's torrent. She held his hand tightly and started walking towards car. "The doctor told you not to drive."
"Don't listen to all his demands!" he shouted.

In her mind's eye, her five-year-old grandson was immersed in playing with his cars. All the little boys were obsessed with cars. As a nursery schoolteacher she had tried in vain to change this stereotypical behavior, but all the girls would run to the doll corner or arts and craft table. She was convinced that car mania was in the Y chromosome. She looked at her husband and wondered how she was going to take away the steering wheel from this grownup boy.

She reached for his coat pocket, grabbed the car keys, and before he could protest, sat in the driver's seat and started the car. He meekly got into the passenger side. A brushfire lit her thoughts. All her resolutions vaporized in its blaze. The dark smoke of anxiety started coming from the tail pipe. Her mind went on a rough ride…

Our path was covered with jasmine.
Why did you have to crush those delicate flowers under your feet, turning the path into a barren wasteland?

Still the memory of its fragrance lingered in my mind.
We were reaching for the Milky Way, but now our dreams imploded.
If only I could turn the Amavasya into a full radiant moon.
At the low tides of our separation, I will stand and prevail.
I will always be longed to be a pearl in your mind's shell.

Traffic was horrible coming home because of the evening rush. A report of doctor's visit must be delivered. I reached for the phone to call my daughters... 'The *coming days are going to be difficult ones*'- I uttered those words and suddenly I am exhausted.

***

It is late at night. I lie in my bed- not a wink of sleep. The clock's red numbers are like hot coal. The blackness of the dark room spreads like a cinder. I can't escape the web of my own thoughts. My mind starts wailing, 'Just rip of the bandage and tell everybody about his state of mind.' Nothing will be same again. Morning comes as I open the door and face the world and the rest of life.

***

Next day he got ready to go to work. She begged him not to drive but he would not budge. Her mind was tormented until he came back in the evening. In a few days, his behavior changed. He kept repeating the same action or asking the same question over and over again. He became stone silent when they had company. He would ignore her often and had trouble following her simple instructions. She was extremely puzzled how he was not making any mistakes at the office. He could not get ready to go to the office on time, had a hard time finding his wallet, keys, belt, handkerchief, etc. Frustrated, he would shout at her. Until now he had never once raised his voice to her. This new Madhukar was totally unknown to her. She would become frightened by his rage and would start crying feebly. She could not face this his new avatar. She kept forgetting that the illness was making Madhukar into this strange angry person. She started pointing out all his wrong doings. Her scolding provoked him into more anger. Their loud quarrels kept bouncing off the walls. It shattered their lovely home's serenity.

Dr. Nair had told her to bring Madhukar back for a follow-up visit in a month. She was dreading facing his cold manners. The long drive also was not good for her back pain. So after a few weeks she wrote a letter explaining Madhukar's condition to their family practitioner Dr, Vandana Khera. They both liked her a lot and had confidence in her. But when Dr. Khera saw him, she admitted that she was not formally trained to take care of Alzheimer's patient. She would only treat him for his physicals and other simple ailments. Dr. Nair was the best in that field, so she had no other choice but to ignore his bluntness and obey his treatments for Madhukar.

***

June 20, 2010

Swati, Madhukar, and I went to Horseneck Beach to celebrate Father's Day. This was our favorite beach. We had been going there since the girls were little. I jumped in the waves to my heart's content. Dinner was of course of fresh lobsters at our usual restaurant in town. After dinner we went meandering in an Audubon wildlife sanctuary across from the eatery. This was our ritual every time we went to that restaurant.

The sun was still floating high on the horizon, and we decided to go a little further to watch the sunset. That road was new to us, but we could see the beach and parking lot in the distance and knew where our car was. Sunset would be in another 40 minutes, so we had plenty of time. The evening was beautiful with a shell pink sky. Colorful birds added more magic to the seascape. The blue waves were alluring. Most of the sunbathers had gone and the solitude was soothing. The tall grass was gently swaying and shimmering gold. Red winged black birds were resting on the feathery tips of the grass. A great heron meditated far away. It was so enchanting that I was immersed in my own world until I came to a rock wall. I knew climbing those rocks would make Madhukar's day complete. Madhukar and Swati were walking ahead of me. I as usual the last car of the train. The rock wall was a little difficult to climb, so I hollered at Swati to hold my hand.

Then Madhukar suddenly stopped and turned around. I was pleased to think that he still cared for my wellbeing and was going to help me up. Alas, that was not the case. "Jyoti there is no way out. The road ends here. We are lost," he quivered.

"Raja, look, there is the beach beyond this wall. Our car is parked there. We are really not that far," I tried to console him. But he was not convinced. He got very scared. Swati showed him her cell phone, "Daddy, don't worry we are not lost. Plus, we can always call somebody for help if needed."

"Who would you call? There's nobody here. Do you know their number?" anxiety took over him completely.

"911 would come to our rescue. Remember we passed the police station on the road?" I pulled his hand and asked him to help me onto the rocks. I wanted him to feel that he is in control. But my feet froze heavy with the fear that he could not remember how to use a cell phone or call 911 on his own. As the weeks passed, simple things confused him. He could not find solutions. His intellect was losing its ability to solve problems. For a few days he would act completely normal again, which would make me doubt my conclusion about him. But he would soon return to a befuddled state of mind.

***

Deep in my heart, the worry was constant and started affecting my rationality also. I started forgetting simple chores of the day. I became worried that I might be walking on the same path as Madhukar.

Our family doctor assured me, "This is a well-known phenomenon of care takers, Jyoti. Worries and emotional demands put a lot of burden on the brain, the brain compensates by only remembering the essential matters and letting go of all else. Stop agonizing. You do not have Alzheimer's. But I did notice that you have lost lot of weight, and I am concerned about your stress levels. How about if I prescribe you something?"

I told her confidently, "With God's grace I have found Yoga-Vedanta philosophy, which gives me a lot of support and helps me understand my journey in life. But if I ever feel the need for a tranquilizer, I will not hesitate to ask you for help." Luckily, I never had to do that. I counted my blessings again and again for the strength Devi had given me.

I found out that the Alzheimer's association helps caregivers as well as the patients. That knowledge should have come from Dr. Nair, but he was only Madhukar's doctor, not mine. So I went to the local support group of the Alzheimer's Association. Listening to other caregiver's horrible stories, I became even more frightened. I did not want to hear about the bleak future. I assured myself that Madhukar was not like that. He was still able to manage his everyday care and go to work, so I stopped going.

But I did attend some workshops which helped me a lot, although the workshops only gave us a manual of physical care, some practical knowledge, and some scientific data. It was like *Para* and *Apara Vidyas*[26] Their curriculum had nothing on spirituality or faith. I strongly believe that there is an unknowable Shakti in this universe; some people call it God or Goddess. I needed to recognize the essential of that Shakti. Then only I would be able to tread the difficult torrent and go across.

***

Her daughters were her solid support. She was so grateful for having them by her side. They were the Goddess's boon to her. One day Chitra took over Daddy's care entirely so Jyoti could go to an

---

[26] Para and Apara Vidya: 'the higher knowledge' is Para Vidya- to learn the Self or the Ultimate Truth i.e. transcendental knowledge. The lower knowledge' is Apara Vidya, consists of all textual knowledge.

important workshop 50 miles away. It was going to be a long day for all of them.

The speaker Joan's husband was diagnosed when he was only 45 years old. Listening to Joan's struggles, Jyoti felt ashamed of her own fatigue. Where did Joan get that courage, she wondered. Jyoti was getting tired of being the person with the heavy load on her shoulders. She decided to change her mindset. She had read many books on Alzheimer's monstrous grip. The day after Joan's lecture, she recognized all the signs that had been mentioned so far. Madhukar had over 90% of the symptoms. Still Joan said that everybody acts differently, and you can't just go by the book. Jyoti started going back to the support group of caregivers. She began heart to heart dialogues with the caregivers and started helping them as much as she could.

There was no cure yet found for Alzheimer's. But she was not going to give up. She would leave no stone unturned. She started showering Madhukar with all the remedies that she came across from the latest research. Turmeric was always the main spice in her cooking ever since she could remember. Recommendations from the talk shows included coconut oil, lavender aromatherapy, sunbathing, etc. If a *Sadhu* had given her a *kala ganda*, black thread, as a talisman, she who was never a believer of that path. But now she would have believed in its power. Now everything had changed. She was so desperate, that she would not have hesitated to tie any amulet around Madhukar's wrist.

The workshop was over. After this emotionally draining day, she could not wait to go home to her beloved. This was the first time she had left him in somebody else's care, never mind that it was his own daughter. She was worried. Poor Chitra; perhaps it had been too much for her. She hoped he had been well-behaved. She became ever more restless. Her mind was entrapped by unending questions. To get out of that whirlpool, she reached for whatever CD her hand first grabbed. The music started with Geeta Dutt's melodious voice.

'Vaktane kiya kya hasi sitam ... tum rahe na tum ham rahe na ham ...Time brings to us such a sweet pleasure of pain ... You are not yourself and neither am I ... our longing hearts come together as if

we were never apart… No sooner than the journey has begun, we are drifting… We have set out. Where to? I do not know… there's no path in sight! What do we seek? I even don't know.'

She was glad to hear her favorite song from the movie Kagajake Phool after so many years. It still made her heart soar. It was like a precious seed, rooted deep down in her heart since her childhood. She adored Geeta Dutt. Her mind went spinning along with the CD and brought her to memories of her sweet childhood.

Where have those golden days gone? Some of her childhood friends had had all the riches, like a fridge, a car, fancy clothes. It didn't matter to her a bit. Her Aai and Dada's boundless love was plenty to cover all her needs. Her Dada never said no to her for anything but of course, she never asked for much. Dada never approved of Bollywood movie songs. She would turn the small radio on sneakily when he was not at home. Shubhi her classmate had 'His Master's Voice' - a huge gramophone. Whenever she visited Shubhi with other friends, they would surround it and soak in all the newest songs. That was the only time she had wished that her Dada could have afforded such a device. After she was married, she mentioned that memory to Madhukar once. When they came to Decatur, Madhukar surprised her with a record player. She was spellbound. Next day she drove 40 miles to Champaign-Urbana, the university town where there was one Indian store. She bought Geeta Dutt's records, and the next few days her apartment was floating with melodies, 'Vaktane kiya kya'…

"Aaji, what this?" Jeevan was puzzled when he saw that LP record in the upstairs storage room decades later. How technology has changed.

***

He had been taking statins for Cholesterol many years per his endocrinologist's advice. Recently when she was on her Google quest, she read that the long-term use of statins can cause memory loss. Immediately she called his Endocrinologist and he agreed on the side effect. She was furious. Knowing Madhukar's current state of mind why did he not stopped the treatment? Why was she the one who had to point it out to him? She had also read that diabetes can cause depression, so she took Madhukar to a psychiatrist. She wanted to save Madhukar from embarrassment, so she wrote the doctor a letter in advance, explaining Madhukar's condition and behavior. She was hoping that he would give Madhukar some supportive counseling. She decided to stay in the room to give Madhukar some comfort.

The psychiatrist started his assessment. His harsh manners shocked her. He was treating Madhukar as a criminal and started interrogating him very cruelly. Instantly she knew she would not stay another moment in that room. Next day she consulted their family physician Dr. Khera who prescribed a mild sedative to calm Madhukar down. It worked like a miracle. His bouts of yelling and being aggressive definitely lessened. She also started having a visiting nurse, Joyce, came to the house once a month. Not only did she help Madhukar, but her kind nature and guidance helped Jyoti tremendously as well. She kept assuring Jyoti that Madhukar's odd behavior, his confused mind his shouting, all would calm down eventually. She prepared Jyoti for the coming future.

***

March 6, 2012

The other day when Jyoti went to pick up dinner from their regular pizzeria, the owner asked why her husband had not come instead, as was usual? She told him about Madhukar's illness without hesitation. Nowadays she could easily mention his Alzheimer's diagnosis even to complete strangers. After such confessions she would feel so light, having shed the extra tons of a heavy burden. Her eyes stayed dry. After dropping Madhukar off at Chitra's home, she went to an evening workshop. The place was closed, and she realized she had gotten the date mixed up. A selfish thought entered her head - *why not go home and spend the evening quietly?* She was stunned at her heartlessness.

"I am on my way, how is Daddy?" Guiltily, she called Chitra right away and told her about the wrong date.

"Aai, why don't you just go home and spend two hours in peace and quiet?" She was surprised by Chitra's request. Did Chitra read my mind? Remorse started poking at her. Chitra insisted that Jyoti should go home and relax. She awkwardly followed her daughter's advice.

On the way home she started making a priority list of all the chores that were left undone since the morning. Suddenly she felt hungry. There were always snacks at the workshops, so she had not planned any dinner that night. She was always careful to take Madhukar's diabetes into consideration when cooking: low carbs, no sugar, high protein. She had learned over the last three decades how to make him balanced and tasty meals, and his doctor always praised her for his controlled sugar levels. It was a balancing act. If he had rice, then no roti. Poor Madhukar, he had never complained about the dietary restrictions. She herself would end up eating the same.

When she reached home, she opened the freezer and hungrily took out frozen dal and roti. Her *thali* was complete with a side dish of homemade *dahi* and lemon pickle, her Aai's special recipe. She didn't have to feed Madhukar, nor wipe away the spills and spits. She wouldn't have to monotonously answer his unending questions. She lit the candle at the kitchen table, turned on *Vishwmohan Bhat's veena* on the CD player, and started her meal without interruption. Raga Puriya mixed more flavors to her comfort food. pulling her into a rare peaceful Vishwa.

December 25, 2012

Three snowstorms one after another suspend the habitat.
Abandoning the birds at the feeders.
Strolls are not possible on these slippery sidewalks.
My mind has frozen like a buried garden.
The gloomy horizon is threatening.
The sky hangs with a deep darkness.
Branches etch in the empty hollows.

Skeletons of the trees- dance wildly in the gusts.
My arteries tighten under the tyrant Old Man Winter's grip.
Layers of black slush thick on both sides.
The road becomes narrower.
I cannot not stay in my lane.
And the decaying road gently reminds me.
The path is not mine alone.
I must share it with fellow travelers.

It was the season of giving and sharing. Colorful lights gleamed in the windows on this Christmas eve, their soft twinkling briefly warmed my frozen mind. My eyes wandered far away. Snow covered the meadow, flapping a white flag of peace. Suddenly I remember another Natal eve with a beautiful purple sky, when Madhukar and I got engaged. His charm had captivated me.

Where has that charismatic personality gone? It shattered into thousands of pieces! Now our dialogues have ceased. Madhukar hardly talks now. He was always doing social work. Due to his talkative nature and ever-readiness to rescue someone in need, he made friends easily. No job was more important than stopping to help fix a flat tire or advising a colleague about investments. He was very social in our new community when we first moved there, but lately I had noticed that he started avoiding people's gaze whenever we went for our evening walks. He would not even greet them or acknowledge them.

When he would hurriedly walk ahead, I pointed it out to him, and he would simply justify his actions, "Well, you talk to them, so the matter is settled." These were very awkward situations for me, and I would find some meek excuse for his behavior and rush to catch up with him.

After a few days of this pattern I gently requested, "Madhukar, at least pause a little bit. If you don't want to say anything, you can simply wave or smile; even a nod would be ok. Otherwise it looks very rude and I know you are never rude to anybody. Please try, Raja."

"Jyoti, I am afraid that I might make a mistake by saying something silly. Then people will think I am stupid! So I prefer to stay silent," his voice faltered.

This was the first and last time he ever expressed his fears to me. Alzheimer's patients don't own anything anymore. The disease robs the victims of their selves. How could I ever console him? I gathered my courage together, "Raja, nobody will think like that or ridicule you. They are our friends. They know you well. Please don't think like that, please say whatever comes to your mind."

But his talking diminished more and more. Not only his voice vanished but his laughter and smiles too. His silence exploded chaos in my mind, suffocating me with loneliness. Sometimes the teacher in me would be eager to school him but then I would remember to be my own student. Instead of prompting or challenging him I would start new life lessons, to adjust my own way of thinking. We were on our evening stroll when Nora came towards us with her dog Tony. Madhukar loved animals and would always pat the neighborhood dogs and play with them. The love was mutual. Tony was always jumping and licking Madhukar joyfully. But today nothing like that happened. Madhukar didn't pat Tony, nor did Tony approach him. Did the dog sense his sickness?

Nora turned to me and asked, "Jyoti, how is he doing?"

It bothered me that Nora did not acknowledge Madhukar directly.

"Why don't you ask him?" the words spilled out of my mouth and Nora obediently repeated the same question to him. To my surprise, Madhukar halted. His head was down, and he didn't look at Nora directly, but he nodded to her. I thought I even saw a little glimpse of a smile on his face. I was thrilled by his response. It meant that he understood her question. This was enough for my hungry heart. But I realized how deep this illness had rooted in him now. I made a pact to myself not to question his behavior anymore but to love him deeply and with all the support I could provide.

When a person is physically bedridden people come to visit the patient. When the patient is counting his last breaths, there is always a long line of friends and waiting to see him. At that point patient is not even aware of his visitors, so what's the use? Alzheimer's does not show any of the physical symptoms in the beginning, so people don't bother to visit them. Very few of our friends came to see Madhukar when they heard about his illness. I used to feel so sad. Maybe others were afraid of how to respond to him? I accepted it finally that everybody has priorities and their own lives to live and that not visiting didn't mean they didn't care.

***

October 2013

Her favorite month October had arrived. Soon it would be Diwali. The Rangoli of colorful leaves in the backyard, the paper lantern, swayed gently on fond memories of Diwali. Normally joy burst like fireworks. Madhukar had always bought her a gift of precious jewels on *Padawa*-the traditional Marathi day for husbands and wives to celebrate each other on the new moon. Even though his negativity was growing like a wild weed, she teased him playfully, "Raja, what gift will you give me this year?

"You don't allow me to drive, so then how can I go out to buy a gift?" he frowned.
"Raja, I don't need any material gift!"

She hurriedly scribbled a few lines on a notepad and stuffed it into his hands.

"How about a love letter like we used to write in our Marriage Encounter group? Or that you used to send me when I was in India?"

She didn't want to pressure him, but she was impatient to see his beautiful handwriting again. She left him alone and fiddled around the house pretending to do chores. She snuck a glance at him, but he was just sitting there holding the pen. She felt renewed pain, recalling that just a few days back it was equally hard for him to sign the form at the bank. A long time passed in stillness and she was giving up but suddenly to her surprise he began writing.

"My dearest Jyoti, not only do I love you, but I adore you more and more every day."
– Madhukar

She read his note greedily and then embraced him excitedly as if she had her old Raja back. All the fancy rings and bracelets that he had given her faded into nothing compared to this priceless and irreplaceable note. She had never celebrated such a wonderful Padwa with him before. Somewhere she heard Barbra Streisand singing, *"And I do anything to get you into my world and hold you within. It's a right I defend, over and over again."* The whole day she was gliding into a beautiful sensation of their everlasting love…

Rangoli that connected the dots of happiness. All the pantyas that flicker disappeared long time ago. But she was glad that the buds of their sweet memories would blossom always as her finger's snap.

She started painting on her mind's canvas, many more qualities of his persona… *Madhukar gave me so much in our life together, and he still keeps giving more. I thought I had all the facets of my diamond; little did I know he had tied the precious jewel into my sari! How was I so blind not to see it?*

***

After our marriage, when he had seen my parent's closeness, he had said hopefully, "Jyoti, if our relationship is like that of your Aai and Dada, then we will have a successful marriage!"

Every couple tries to be very loving and add romance towards each other when they are newly married. But once the honeymoon is over, the reality of life's responsibility hits and the romance gets overridden. They start taking each other for granted. The husband is buried in office work and is always so tired when he returns home in the evenings. The wife has no choice, no matter how high a position she holds in her career. Her housework is never finished, and she can never retire. We were no exception to this rule.

But one thing was always there - our heart-to-heart chats. Madhukar was initially inclined to remain quiet when it came to express his personal feelings. Over the years I learned to hear the words within his silence. Still, in the beginning, I had no idea what he was thinking about; he had a hard time communicating. It was always a guessing game when he was quiet or became melancholy. After many months I was beginning to understand this loving clam that I was married to.

At our wedding ceremony, the priest had tied a sacred thread around us. It had seemed so flimsy and delicate then, but now I know it was no ordinary strand. Over the years that strand became stronger with our nurturing love and devotion towards each other. But now all that is becoming foggy. Without being aware of his silent teachings in the past, now I stumble upon them constantly. We were always aware of and grateful for our true solidarity and companionship. We were each other's mirrors. While walking on the smooth path with him I never had the slightest idea how much he had given me. Now that this cruel illness has swallowed him, I realize his true value. I have lost a dear friend. It makes my heart bleed that I won't be ever able to tell him my gratitude.

***

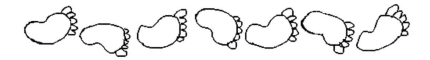

Being deeply loved by someone gives you strength, while loving someone deeply gives you courage. - Lao Tzu

Where should I start? One can never count the shells on the beach, the waves in the ocean, the whispering leaves of an oak tree, the blades of grass covering the meadow, the stars in the night sky. Our life was full of a thousand happy memories, blossoming at each moment. How can one measure the joy? The equation of our marriage would always be $1+1 = 1$.

"You are such a brilliant, smart intelligent man! How did you ever say yes to me, who is so ordinary compared to your accomplishments?" I had nervously asked him on the very first night of our wedding.

"Jyoti, when I first saw you, I made up my mind to marry only you! I was extremely impressed with your daring to choose a field outside of the norms. An artist cannot create anything unless she is also intelligent. Jyoti, did you know mathematics is also an art?" I was astonished to hear his explanation. Aai and Aba had fully supported me in my pursuit of art, so Dada reluctantly allowed me to join J.J. School of Arts. But until now nobody had ever worshiped my creativity with such heartfelt admiration. I was overwhelmed and thanked God over and over again for giving me such an appreciative soulmate. His arrival in my life opened a door for my muse.

I remember one incidence vividly. I was in Dadar, visiting Aai Dada just a week after we were married. Madhukar was hovering over me like a bee. Those were the heady days of newly found love. He handed me a math textbook and asked me to keep it safe. I dutifully locked it in the locked cabinet. We returned to Dombivili by local train as we were disembarking, he reached for the book, questioning, did you open it?"

"No," I shook my head.

He winked at me, "Nobody ever bothers to look at math books, so I knew that our cash would be safe."

He flipped all the pages as if they were playing cards; inside was hidden his entire salary for the week. I laughed, amused by his cleverness, and at the same time pleased that he had given all his money in my hands. From that day on he trusted me with money matters and never once asked me for an account of my spending.

Madhukar truly loved my parents as if his own. I used to get very homesick for them when I was new in America. In that longing, once I barely mentioned, "Wouldn't it be nice if they could visit us here?" I knew neither Dada nor we could afford the expensive airline tickets. But later when we had more savings, Madhukar remembered and bought them the tickets. I could not thank him enough!

Two days after we were married, we had gone by train to pay our respects to his eldest uncle in Solapur, about 300 miles away from Bombay. We had to change our compartment at the last minute. The train was about to leave, so as we were running to our reserved compartment, suddenly Madhukar realized that he had left his Nikon camera in the previous compartment. Then again, he started running back, me panting, trying to catch up with him. He totally forgot that I was with him. I wondered why I didn't take his aunt seriously when she had warned me about his absent mindedness?

We got down at Solapur station. There were some horse buggies, waiting for the customers. I signaled him and started walking towards the carriage …

"Jyoti, horse ride through this traffic will take too much time," but he followed me obediently. My mind started galloping with the horses. The road turned and excitedly I yelled at the horseman to stop the carriage. Madhukar's eyebrows raised. I pointed at a beautiful branch of a flowering tree, bending like a dancer's arm. Silently I glanced at the camera in his hands and pointed my chin, gesturing him to take a picture of that branch. He got down, the frown changing into a delightful smile. He took few photos from different angles, under my direction.

"Now can we go?" his affectionate gaze told me all over again that I have indeed found my Raja. His cooperative act made me euphoric. This how our artful, heartfelt seven steps journey truly began under that blossoming branch.

Soon Sankranti arrived. As per tradition, a newly bride is decorated with ornaments made out of halwa, a sugar crystal candy. All the ladies begged me to say an *Ukhana*, another silly custom in my opinion. It was a chance for the newlyweds to say each other's names aloud. Normally, it was considered impolite for a bride to use her husband's name in public. So putting his name into a clever rhyming poem was her only chance. I was irritated, but then suddenly I heard:

'One beautiful evening blossomed in a flowering blue sky, while Shubhangi mesmerized my eye.'

Madhukar's poem melted all of my irritation away. Per yet another tradition, Madhukar's aunt changed my name to Shubhangi when we were married. He had asked me how I felt about it, and I guess when you are in love, you don't have any sense, so I full heartedly agreed to the name change, which was traditional back then in Indian culture. But he never ever actually called me Shubhangi; to him I was always Jyoti.

Madhukar's motto was to enjoy life fully. Every time we moved into a new house; he would urge me to change the décor according to my taste right away. "Don't wait to improve the house only when it's time to sell it. Let's enjoy it now."

He was my handyman and fix-it all man. When we moved to Norton, I chose a very different color, a dull olive green for our living room. I would always use daring colors on the walls that nobody else would try but this time I was a little hesitant about my choice.

He smiled, "Jyoti don't worry, if you don't like it then I will paint over it with another color of your choice." He never interfered when it came to my interior decoration.

I always was amused by his daily puns and jokes; sometimes even though he was hilariously funny, I would tease him, "I am not laughing at your joke, Mister, I am laughing at you."

One time we were walking in a mall in McKinney. He went on his own while I stopped to rest. As he returned, there was a little twinkle in his eyes. Before I could inquire, he said with a chuckle, "Today I finally found out Victoria's secret."

I rolled my eyes, "What were you doing in there, Madhukar?"

"I didn't have to go inside; it was all in an open display in the window," he protested.

His command of languages was incredible. He was fluent in English, Hindi, Sanskrit, Marathi, French, and a little Italian and Russian. When we used to travel abroad, he would pick up the local language right away. When playing *Antakshari*, he would instantly translate Bollywood Hindi songs into Marathi and sing them in the same tune, both amusing and confusing everyone.

Later his command of Sanskrit came very handy when he started a hobby of officiating weddings, coming of age thread ceremonies, vastu shanti for new homes, and many other religious rituals. Seeing and helping him in those rituals, I learned a lot. Once I also was able to perform a 'Satyanarayana Puja' at my friend's house in Dallas.

Even though his childhood was scarred by extreme deprivation, he was never bitter towards his parents. He inherited his father's devotion for the *Dnyaneshwari* and *Bhagavad Gita* and could recite verses by heart. I had brought his father's *Dnyaneshwari* with me from Dombivili. Madhukar and I would read both of those books together on a regular basis throughout our lives, a memory that I am so grateful for. Our common interest in Indian philosophy was indeed a boon for both of us.

Some of his favorite slogans were: *'Never give up.' 'Don't accept defeat.' 'Always try something new.' 'Why be normal? Normal is boring.' 'Once you give a donation to a someone, never ask how he/she is going to spend it; that is none of your business.' 'This country has given me so much. We owe so much to this land.'* He was stubbornly patriotic and very much a democrat. So extremely so that he would not even drive on the George Bush Highway in Dallas, even though the toll was less, and the speed was faster than on other routes!

Phalnitakar Aaji was very dear to me and was one of my favorite and most admired ladies. She was not related to me, but we called her Aaji out of respect. She had invited me for *Shrawani Shukrawar*, a special celebration of married women. Since Madhukar was home, she had invited him to come along too. She did *Arti* to me and started bowing down when I abruptly stopped her from doing so. "Aaji, what are you doing? I should be the one bowing to you for your blessings!" She innocently blurted, "Jyoti you have been married to Madhukar for so long, that's why I bow to you." All she had meant was that she was celebrating my role as wife. I mischievously giggled, agreeing with her that yes indeed I should be honored for putting up with Madhukar all these years. After a feast of delicious homemade *puran polis* (sweet chickpea flour- stuffed rotis), we were returning home.

Suddenly Madhukar asked me, "Jyoti did I take good care of you?" I was puzzled. Where was this coming from? Was he thinking about what Phalnitakar Aaji said to me? I poked him, pretending I was Golde from "The Fiddler on the Roof." "For 25 years, I've washed your clothes, cooked your meals, cleaned your house, given you daughters. After 25 years, why talk about love right now?"

"I was reminiscing about that long-ago Sunday at your parents' home in Dadar, right after our wedding. Your Aai gave me an extra helping of sweet *Shreekhand*. Your cousin *Bhau* pouted because he thought that she didn't give him as much as me. So she answered him while smiling at me, *'Dear Bhau, Madhukar is going to take care of your Jyoti tai from now on.'* Oh, I was petrified to hear those expectations. Nobody had ever expressed so directly to me my lifelong responsibilities to you, my new wife… "

"Jyoti, tell me the truth." He avoided looking directly at me and kept his eyes on the road, his left hand clutching the steering wheel. I laced my fingers in his other hand, "See if you can feel my answer through my touch."

***

Madhukar had a knack for planning for our future. He did our financial planning very thoughtfully and with great vision. He was very keen on making sure we would be self-sufficient in our old age. Every Sunday he would sit at his computer to see where the market was heading. He urged me many times to sit and learn, but I didn't pay much attention to his begging and avoided it with some excuse. That was not my cup of tea!

I didn't want to have one more chore added to my list. He was completely unaware that things like toothpaste, paper towels, shaving cream, etc. ran out and had to be replenished. So I took in charge of all the other responsibilities of our everyday living, and that was enough. I paid the monthly bills and balanced the checkbook. Not only that, but when it was time to buy a new car or house, Madhukar would nudge me into the bargaining because he was too shy to do so.

He always needed a challenge. I remember in our very first house on Michael Road when I designed a wall-to-wall desk for the girls, not knowing anything about carpentry Madhukar nevertheless took the initiative and built it. He enjoyed any kind of hard physical work. After getting some lessons from a local carpenter, he even added a whole new room to the house! And this was before the days of internet and YouTube videos. It always amazed me to see his constant yearning to learn something new.

One day we were going for a ride to look at the beautiful fall foliage. On the road I saw lots of tree stumps. An idea for an unusual base for a coffee table floated in my mind. I told him to stop the car and explained my idea. Before I knew it, one heavy stump was already in our trunk. Then the next two weeks he was so busy sandpapering, varnishing, and changing the ordinary stump into a beautiful table base that he forgot his hunger and thirst. That coffee table became not just the center of our living room but was always a piece of admiration by the people who came to visit us. Forty years later I still have it.

Madhukar always tried to live passionately and in style. 'If I eat, it will be always with *ghee*, or else I would rather go hungry' was his motto. Whatever hobbies he pursued he would reach the top with that attitude. I often felt homesick for my childhood beach in Dadar, but my love affair with water truly began at the pond behind our Michael Road house. Its water lilies, swans and Canadian geese were so enchanting for a city girl like me. The pond taught me how to enjoy all four seasons. In the winter, the pond would offer a great skating rink for all the people in town. Their colorful sweaters fluttering like butterflies brought spring in the middle of winter. I would sit, my nose stuck to our glass window and watch them endlessly. But with Madhukar it was a whole different story. One day he exclaimed, "*Saalye*-Those rascals come and skate on my backyard pond? I guess I will have to learn how to skate too." So at age 40 this young man decided to put on skates and join them, dragging me along. After falling on my butt a couple of times, I gave up and decided to watch the excitement from inside my warm home with a cup of hot chocolate in my hand. Madhukar also fell a lot, but the words "I can't do it" were not in his vocabulary. Father and daughters had a ball skating side-by-side.

Madhukar went on bike for a long trip when he had lived in Pune, a city famous for loving bicycling. He would take Swati and Chitra on long rides. My story was different. I never rode on the busy streets of Bombay. I used to rent a bike for 25 annas per hour. Our servant Ramchandra would come with me to Shivaji Park and hold the bike so this princess could get on it and start peddling. So I never learned how to get on and off a bike by myself. When Madhukar found this out, he taught me how, making me practice fifty times until I was very capable. He was a tough teacher. Then every evening our whole family, a cycling *barat*, would ride around in the neighborhood. Over the course of a few months I began to enjoy bicycling. Later when the girls were in college, just the two of us visited Martha's Vineyard by ferry, bringing our bikes. Swati and Madhukar always rode in front of the runners during the Boston Marathon, back when that was allowed. They also participated in roundtrip100 mile bike-a-thon fundraising for Multiple Sclerosis research from Amherst to New Hampshire. In Swati's words, 'it was uphill both ways.' Madhukar subsequently participated in many other bike-a-thons.

His adventurous nature was sometimes scary. We all had got a taste of his challenging nature on a trip to Kashmir, in the Himalayas. We were on the banks of the Zelam River. The water was violently turbulent with whirlpools. Our car driver stopped at the water's edge to watch the raging whitewater. There was a suspension "bridge "(calling it a bridge was generous) that consisted of a few ropes tied together for the army to use. Madhukar the daredevil went skipping on to the bridge before we knew it, trying to cross the river. There was a lot of gaps between the woven steps. One could easily miss and fall into the rough water beneath. Seeing him there on the dangling rope, my heart skipped several beats. Everybody from the group was urging him to come back, but he just kept moving further. Chitra was in third grade and Swati in fifth grade at the time. They got really scared and started crying. My elderly aunt Akka also requested him to return to shore, but he smilingly ignored us all. "*Madhukar, if not for me, at least return for your young daughters' sakes. Don't forget you are a father. If you fall and drown, I will never forgive you for depriving your girls of their daddy. That's my final warning.*" Thank Goddess, that message reached him, and he came back safely to shore.

I am so glad that we traveled a lot while we were young. Madhukar loved to plan our trips, making sure to visit where normal tourists would not bother to go or to know about much less even. Our agenda always included local universities, botanical gardens, farmer's markets, and of course art museums. While working at MITRE Corporation, he was selected to present at an important defense conference in Monterey, California. We decided to make that trip into a little vacation. For two days we enjoyed being in Monterey's 'high society'. Seeing Lamborghinis crowding the parking lots made his day. On the morning of the day that he was to present his paper, he had a little free time, and decided to roam around bit. I packed a nice breakfast for us to eat on the beach. The fragrance of orange blossoms was intoxicating. Deer prancing on the beach added an extra charm to the sunny morning. After a few hours I reminded him about the conference.

"Don't you want to prepare a little bit for your presentation?

He didn't have any previous experience about the defense industry, and I was getting a little nervous on his behalf.

"Jyoti, why are you stressed? I'm the one presenting the paper!"

I don't know how long we meandered around. I again reminded him, and finally we headed back to the hotel. He had just enough time to change into formal attire and dash out of the door. Thank goodness, the conference was downstairs in the same hotel. In the late afternoon he returned, "Jyoti, what's the plan? Where do you want to go now?" he said, not mentioning the presentation at all.

In the evening after dinner, I asked him finally, a little timidly, "So how was it? Did you do ok?"
He replied nonchalantly, "Oh, everything went fine. My paper was awarded first prize.'

To be fair, absentmindedness always went hand in hand with his extraordinary intellect. We would often have to remind him that the girls and I were waiting for him for dinner. He would always find some excuse to be late, and would finally come downstairs, a book in his hand. He was distracted, reading while eating, and half the time he would not pay any attention to what was on his plate unless, God forbid, something was wrong with my cooking. I would get so annoyed. But later on when it was just the two of us in our empty nest, he started giving me compliments. Not only that, but once in a while he would confess that I was winning in the game of love, conquering him entirely.

I could write a book just about his absent-mindedness. If I had not chosen his outfit and laid his clothes out for him every day, he might even have gone to work in his birthday suit! Sometimes he would wear two different colored socks to work (this was long before it became fashionable to wear unmatched clothing). To solve that problem, I started buying socks of all the same color.

He was adamant about bringing lunch from home, with the excuse that it was a waste of time to have to go back and forth to the cafeteria at work. So every day I had to pack his lunch. I used to put some love notes or Jasmine flowers in his lunch box. I was hoping it would add a little extra flavor to his busy days. I should have known better than to hope he would even acknowledge these little gestures. Finally I got fed up, so one day I put my love note inside his sandwich, hoping that at least now he would have to notice it. In the evening when he returned, there was no comment from him. Losing my patience. I asked him how his sandwich had tasted.

"Oh, it was fine but there was some kind of paper in it that I ended up chewing." After that I gave him plain boring lunches without any extra spices.

Once we watched '*Bagban*', a Bollywood movie starring Amitabh Bachchan and Hema Malini. In the film they were married for 25 years yet were still behaving like lovebirds! I was puzzled and a little envious of that couple. Well, that only happens in movies, I tried to console myself and went to bed that night still thinking about it. The next day I decided to play a joke on my darling husband by following the heroine's daily routine. She would get all dressed-up just before her husband came back from the office every evening. Then she would greet him holding a tea tray in her hand, which she would later serve him in the garden while they had a nice chat. I got all dressed up just like her, putting on one of the beautiful silk saris that Madhukar had given me a long time ago. I heard Madhukar's car in the garage. We had a sterling silver tea set that my Aai had given to me as part of our wedding gift. Tray in hand and holding my breath, I poised near the entrance as Madhukar walked in.

"Hello darling!" I cooed, trying my best not to laugh.
He was startled and looked at me dumbfounded, a large question mark spreading all over his face.
"What is this? Why are you standing here like this, Jyoti?" and with that he simply walked inside. I got no hugs like Amitabh had

bestowed on Hema. After that I tried awfully hard to squelch my romanticism, but my heart wouldn't allow it.

***

Madhukar always measured his sugar before bedtime and took his insulin dose accordingly. One night, I called him for his snack and a glass of warm milk to last him through the night. I waited for a while for his answer. So I loudly yelled, "Madhukar, where are you?" Still no response. I figured he must be in the library (read: bathroom) and I went to knock on the door. To my surprise the bathroom was empty. So I thought he was upstairs in his office, his eyes glued to the computer, and ears not working as usual. So I went upstairs stamping my feet, but he wasn't there either. I began to worry now. Where could he be? Did he go to sleep? So I decide to check the bedroom. The bed was still made. There was a cool gust coming so I went around the bed to close the window. I was confused to see light coming from under the bed. I bent down. I saw my husband all squeezed under the bed on his stomach. He was holding a table lamp in his one hand and in other hand was his cell phone.

"Madhukar, what are you doing under there?!'"

"I am testing the alarm on my new blackberry. I want to make sure it is working."

"But why do you have to be under the bed?" I was losing my patience.

"Oh... I could not find any other sockets in the bedroom," he sheepishly replied.

That was around 2011, when he had started consulting at A123. In a week he was going to China for a business trip. At that point, I didn't care if his phone was working or not, but I sure was alarmed about his common sense/sanity.

"My dear husband, Bombay University's gold medalist, Professor Madhukar Vishwanath Joshi, with a Doctorate in Statistics from the Case Western Institute of Technology, did you even look?"

I held my palms together and mockingly bowed to him while I pointed to about eight sockets in the bedroom and adjoining bathroom and hallway.

"Oh. I didn't see them," he replied, still looking sheepish. I started laughing hilariously. When I have my dear Raja side by me, I do not need to go to any comedy clubs!!!

His and my birthdays were just a week apart, and his birthday even came first but he would still manage to forget my birthday each year. Then I would have a temper tantrum. As our daughters got older, they would always remind their father, "Daddy, buy flowers for Aai today."

"Why?" he would ask them innocently. But he would bring me surprise gifts whenever he felt like it. He would always encourage me to pursue my art. He took time to learn the art of making frames long time ago. As soon as he saw my finished painting, there was not much vocal praise from him but instantly he would secure my painting in a homemade frame. When I had solo exhibitions, he would move the paintings to the exhibit hall and of course hang them perfectly on the walls. Joy and pride overflowed on his face.

When we were engaged, I was worried that I didn't know him enough to marry him. But finally I came to see his true identity and his honest love towards me, hidden in all the facets of his character. His zest for life always shone. His unspoken words and teachings… all these gifts would last for me until our next seven lives together.

***

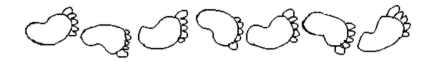

The atman is imperishable, and it pervades the whole universe. - Sri Krishna in Bhagavad Gita

October 13, 2013

I decided to give an unusual gift to myself. The Vedic period (c. 1500 – c. 500 BCE) in India was very progressive. It was very common for the girls also to have *Munj- a thread ceremony* [27], one of the sixteen samskaras in Hindu religion. I had wanted to do that for my girls, but I it slipped my mind when they were growing up. Jeevan, our grandson was eight years old now, the perfect age for a Muja. I knew Madhukar would have loved to officiate, but unfortunately, he hardly spoke anymore. My stubborn mind still believed that sometimes he was able to observe and understand what was going on around him. So I decided to do Jeevan's Munj. I tried my best to teach him nearly 30 shlokas, Sanskrit religious and spiritual poems. At age three he could easily chant the 'Gayatri Mantra' fluently. I tried to explain him the true meaning of Munj to his age level. He liked the idea and wanted to perform the ceremony.

All the ladies in the house were involved in the ceremony. I officiated, Chitra performed the rituals, and Swati whispered a guru mantra in Jeevan's ears. Mark took over the very important task of taking pictures. We made sure that Madhukar was sitting comfortably in the corner where he could watch; Holly, his caretaker, was there with him so that we could focus on the ceremony without having to worry about him.

---

[27] Munj, or thread ceremony- in which a guru draws a child towards knowledge and initiates the second birth of the young mind and spirit. It is similar to a Bar or Bat Mitzvah.

Guru Purnima had happened just a week ago, and I had been missing my Aai, my first Guru. The scriptures always say before you begin any rituals you should bow to your Guru for blessings. As I started the ceremony, before even I could think of my parents or other spiritual gurus, I quickly went to Madhukar and held his hands. I made sure that he felt my touch and then I humbly bowed to him. I wondered if he still remembered that long ago, I confessed to him that he was my soulmate and husband, but most importantly he was my guru.

Whenever we watched Bengali movies, and the wife would touch her husband's feet in the morning before starting her day. I would always object furiously, arguing that husband and wife are equals. I would never do that to you, Madhukar, I would tease him. Sometimes I would only bow to him in mockery, to salute this perpetually absent-minded professor. But that day I bowed to him in earnest, with all my gratitude. He will always be my guru. That is the ultimate truth. I have tried to digest all the philosophy to learn about the real I, but, in the end, Madhukar is the one who was guiding me through his cruel illness to find the quest of the soul, Atman. Now I know why mother Kunti asked to Krishna to give her a life full of sorrows/difficulties; only then would she remember to worship him constantly.

***

December 19, 2013

They went for a walk on the golf course behind their condo community. She remembered that first Sunday long ago when he pampered her by taking to the Country Club in Decatur. This city girl had never seen so much sap-green color blanketing the earth. She bent down and touched the soft grass. He was amused by her reaction. They had a lavish breakfast…thick stacks of pancakes with fresh strawberries and blueberries, covered with whip cream, drenched with maple syrup. From then on it became a Sunday ritual. She could still feel the taste of maple syrup on her tongue.

Such a carefree life. While holding on to those comforting memories not letting it go like a baby blanket, she lost herself and stumbled into a little ditch on the ground. She reached out to grab on to a nearby branch, only to feel sharp thorns needling her fingers- at that very moment she saw the red berries hidden inside the shiny green leaves of that holly bush.

Those happy memories trickled away through the drops of red blood… The thorns punctured her delicate fingers. Ignoring her pain, she looked at the red berries, a perfect addition to her pinecone Christmas décor on the fireplace mantel. She always took pride in using nature's abundant treasures. From the corner of her eye, she saw him walking as usual, seven steps ahead of her. Her mind persuaded her, "*It will be just a minute.*"

She stopped and started cutting the thorny branches with her bare hands. When she turned around, he was not there. There was a bend on the road. So, she walked faster to catch up with him. Still she could not see him. Where did he go? She had only lingered at the bush for a moment. He must have taken the other path at the fork, and not their usual one. So, she went on.

the other path, but still could not locate him. Her mind started racing. He knows this golf course, so he can't be that far. She craned her neck to look for him only to see the blue-sky melt in the hills. How could he just disappear?

Then she remembered that at the Alzheimer's workshop, somebody was telling about how his father had gotten lost. She had never given it a thought. She had assumed he would always be walking by her side. Her mouth went dry. All the joy from those berries disappeared and their red color bled in her mind more than those thorns did on her fingers and she began to panic. "He can't get lost, I will never forgive myself," she wailed.

She started running looking for him, asking every person she came across but all of them shook their heads negatively in response. Fifteen minutes passed with no sign of him. The golf course covered so many square miles of rolling hills. It would be impossible to comb all that land with her weak feet. She called her daughter Chitra,

"Should I call the police?"

Chitra calmed her down and started the car to come to her rescue. Jyoti imagined the worst scenario, her mind always so overly imaginative. In the distance she saw a golf cart coming slowly towards her, and she saw a glimpse of something red in it. She thought the redness of the berries had contaminated her eyes too. But as the golf cart came closer to her, she saw him in his red jacket. She had bought that color, so he could easily spot his jacket in the closet, a tip she had learned from the dementia caregivers' workshop.

The golf cart slowed down next to her; she was so relieved to see him safe. She thanked the driver profusely for bringing Madhukar back to her. He looked so innocent, didn't say a word. She wondered if he even knew that he had gotten lost. She wanted to shout at him. *How dared he go without her!* But she controlled herself and held his hand gently to help him get down from the cart.

This incident shook her like an earthquake but also taught her a lesson. I must be very watchful like a hawk who sits on the tall oak tree in our backyard searching for prey. She bit her tongue - *he is not her prey, but Alzheimer's.*

As soon as they came home, she wrote lots of notes – her and daughters' names and numbers, his name and contact info, and his illness. She put one copy in his wallet, one in the car, and one in each of his jackets. She also wrote all the information in permanent ink on the collar of his jackets. Next day she went to the police station and gave them his photo id and other necessary information. Still she did not feel confident. The next few days and weeks went in watching him constantly as if she was his jailer. If she heard a slight noise, she would run to see if he had gotten out of the house.

***

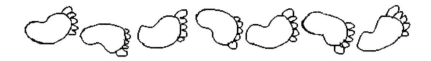

We must let go of the life we have planned, so as to accept the one that is waiting for us. - Joseph Campbell

'When will his calm disposition come back? It has to come back!', she was heartbroken over her loss. She became obsessed to try whatever would make him get better. Her only aim was to pull him out of that dreadful disease. She would overturn every stone around to make him cured.

Mother Earth's beauty had always whispered gently to her like a soothing lullaby in times of stress. From childhood she would always enjoy being in nature; she was grateful for this boon of appreciation, knowing that not everyone had it. There is no healer like nature. They always had gone in the woods behind their house. She started taking him there again, so he could feel calm deep down.

Classical music also has the same power of healing. She used to play particular Indian classical ragas for her yoga students during meditation. Indian classical music would always kindle the creativity in her heart. He was the one who introduced her to western classical. They both were passionate about going to concerts. Classical music constantly resonated in their house. Now she used music as therapy for him at home as well as in the car. She used "Om" CD on for chanting. Whenever somebody entered their *'Whispering Oaks'* house in Framingham, they would say, "Jyoti, your house has some sacred peace!"

She would simply smile and reply,

"That's the effect of *Om*. We always chant that magical Omkar in our Yoga class here."

She had hoped that he would get all better. He would beat all the statistics in the studies and be the exception to the rule of no recovery. But in spite of all of her constant efforts, she was no longer so sure. Lately she started feeling depressed. Her desire to free him from the Chakravyuh[28] of that unconquerable illness was sucking all her energy away and she was losing her motivation. Each morning she would start her day with new hope, but as the sunset came all her shakti would disappear into the darkness of night. She would become very cranky. While trying to calm him down at bedtime, she would lose her own sleep. Head tossing on the pillow she would repeat the prayer in her mind:

'I am the most powerful and strong spirit the Atman. I am the ultimate joy and bliss.

I am the purest soul. I am immortal!!!

I am Malati Deodhar's -my mother's- daughter. I will not give up. I will care of him. Devi, you are his only savior, and I know you are looking after him. Please give me the strength and courage and wisdom to care for him with eternal love.

Veer Savarkar's oath to fight for freedom against the British echoed in her head. *'Ki ghetale vrat na he, amhi andhatene...* We did not take this vow blindly; we knew we would burn in this fire.' Today she could truly comprehend the shloka her Aai taught her when she was hardly 7 years old.

***

It was time to take him to the adult day care center. I asked him to sit on the stairs so I can put the shoes on his foot, as that angle was much easier for my aching back. After I put socks on his feet, I told him to put his foot in the shoe, but he just sat there. I told him again to do it. He moved a bit but again he just sat still. It was getting late. It was very painful when I tried in vain to put his rigid feet in the shoes;

---

[28] Chakravyūha is a military formation used to surround enemies, depicted in the Hindu epic Mahabharata. It resembles a labyrinth or multiple defensive walls.

the arthritis in my wrist was getting worse day by day. Unconsciously I held my breath, getting annoyed. I was about to yell at him for his laziness, *how can you not do such a simple thing?* But I got control of myself and just asked him with a firm voice,

"Madhukar, are your hearing aids not working? Or you are just ignoring me?"

"Jyoti, I can hear you and understand what you are telling me to do, but I just can't do it."

His eyes welling with tears, his lips trembling, and I heard his voice quivering. Like a flash of lightning, it occurred to me that his brain was not able to send the command. He simply does not have the control over it.

'*How in the world could this brilliant man reach this stage? How is he able to face this reality?*'

My eyes opened a dam of gushing tears, and the naked truth stood right there in front of me. God is testing me! I surrendered to that very moment. What is god, after all? She does not live in a temple. Her shakti dwells in all of us.

I realized if I do not have faith in that shakti, -higher power, then there is nothing I can attain in life. Without true surrendering of my ego, it is all in vain.

My parents embedded that teaching in me through their everyday examples. I thanked them again and became indebted to the supreme power. From now on Madhukar is my only true God. "*Raja, don't worry, I am at your service, dear,*" I gently patted on his back. I held his shoes parallel to his feet and succeeded getting them on. Our feet started tapping towards the garage in the same rhythm.

***

May 8, 2011

I did not feel like getting up in the morning. The negative thoughts thickly blanketing me hid my normal chi. I forced myself to do my morning rituals - yoga, pranayama, hoping to bring my mind back to normal.

He was still sleeping. I envied him. I started to rush as usual trying to obey my never-ending list of "*Things to do.*" I let 10 minutes go by, still no sign of him waking up, so I tried to coax him and planted a gentle kiss on his forehead. He did not even stir a bit. Suddenly I got so frightened from his stillness, I my put my ear to his heart. His calm rhythmic breathing made me relax. It had been a long time since he had slept so soundly like that.

I opted to forgo my usual hurry and gave him that luxury to sleep as long as he wanted. He looked so innocent as a baby, so carefree in sound sleep, not a single trace of his confusion or dementia. His calmness gave me hope. Maybe my old Raja is back? I wanted to lock his innocence in my heart. Lately his *moun vrat- vow of silence, was* in full practice. I longed to hear his laughter, his whispers in my ears. Even his monosyllabic responses, "*Hum! Ok!*" would have been welcome. I left him and started getting breakfast ready while listening to the '*Shivoham Shivoham'* bhajan.

In a while he got up and we ate breakfast together calmly. '*Is this the calm before the storm?'* I ignored my mind's grumbles. We left the house for the pool.

The splashes of swimming tried to encourage my mind a bit. But in the next minute I became melancholy and finished my swimming robotically. Usually the whirlpool gave me a relaxing massage. Madhukar, in a daze, was still hovering around the pool, walking in circles. His incessant spinning made me dizzy. His descending state of mind seared me. I tried to console myself that maybe a hot shower would take away all my anguish.

Cathy's swimming class was just over, and all those little wet bodies were out of the pool. They looked like little angels with their white towels flapping around them. I always noticed how good she was with those little kids. Jeevan had loved her class. I rushed to the grid iron gate to get out of the pool area, navigating my way through all the little swimmers. A little girl from Cathy's class came running to the gate, opened the door as if she were rescuing me. "You are getting out of jail now. You're free!" Startled by her words, I stared at her. How did she know my incarceration, the heavy chains of my burden?

***

May 9, 2011

Jeevan came over later on that Sunday afternoon. I could see the fatigue on his face from yesterday's bike-a-thon. Only eight years old he rode for eight miles continuously, collecting the topmost money for the charity. I lay down on the couch next to him to read him a book. Just then Swati arrived as usual. She had been coming every Sunday to help me with Daddy. She also started cuddling. I knew my girls were also incredibly stressed, but they did not talk about their worries in my presence in order to shield me. They chose to deal with their father's illness silently. Her loving touch made me happy. I do not know why, but out of nowhere, I started chanting *Om*. It always released my stress like a magic. I heard Swati's humming Om. Mimicking her, Jeevan also joined our chorus.

The vibrating sound of *Om* started filling the room. Madhukar was taking a nap in the bedroom. He must have been awakened by our chanting. He came to see us. His face was blank. He looked so vulnerable. As he started to go back… Jeevan begged him,

"*Ajoba, please stay.*" Jeevan adores his Ajoba.

"*Daddy, hold my and Aai's hand,*" Swati also urged him.

"*Raja just hold my hand,*" I tried to encourage him also.

Still, he could not comprehend it. Confusion spread all over his face. The dialogue resonated in my mind about when I had told him to put his shoes on. But suddenly a miracle happened. He came near us and held our hands. Our eight hands locked in a loop; Om became complete in a full rhythmic circle of *Nada Brahma*. We could hear his hazy stuttering for few moments and then his mouth just stayed opened without any sound. The power of Om! His face became alive again. Long lost hidden contentment rose on his face. At last my long-lost dear Raja came to visit me, back again just for a blink. My eyes started trickling.

"Why are you crying?" his question shocked me with joy.

Did I really hear him say that? I wanted to pinch myself to make sure it was not a dream. I could have danced all night on his words. How should I answer him?
Dumbfounded, I was trying to find some words!

"Ajoba, Aaji is not crying. She is happy. Those are happy tears," Jeevan came to my rescue.

***

March 2011

He came home from work with bad news; his company was suddenly closing next week. They did not get their grant. Naturally, he was upset, but she was happy to hear the news, actually. She released a quiet sigh of relief. No more long drives to work.

Lately, even little things bothered him. He became agitated by the slightest change. If a leaf moved because of the wind, his mood would be off.

The other day, he could not find the belt that Chitra bought for him. There are about 4 or 5 belts hanging in his closet, but he wanted that particular one. So he became terribly angry. If he had to sit on a different chair at the dining table, he would start fidgeting. She had noticed that if there was a slight change in his routine, he would get very disturbed. From tomorrow on he would be home all day, due to the closing of his company. She resolutely decided to plan his days in the same exact patterns. She remembered from the book that the same routine everyday gives some security to these patients. His comfort was going to be her *dharma* from now on.

"Jyoti wake up. We overslept. It's 2 p.m. in the afternoon!" Madhukar was shaking her fiercely. She was sound asleep for a change and awoke with a jolt. The room was filled with such bright light that it bothered her eyes. How did I sleep so late? She blinked her eyes again and turned towards the clock on her bedside table. It was indeed 2 o'clock. But something was strange. Outside it was still dark. She noticed the full moon peeping into their window. Reality hit her; it was 2 all right, but a.m., not p.m. The bright glow was coming from the lights that Madhukar had turned on all over the house. His sugar measurement kit was opened and placed on his side of the bed, the needle package unopened. Looked like he did not measure his sugar yet. He always measured his sugar only at the kitchen table. He was yelling for nothing. She tried to coax him,

"Raja, it's still night, lets sleep now. Tomorrow morning as usual you can measure your sugar."

He would not budge. She gave him some snacks to distract him. Still he was pacing in the house.

"Let's go back to bed."

One by one she turned off the lights, pointing at the dark sky outside. Still he was not convinced. When they finally went to bed, it was almost 4 AM. He fell asleep right away, but her mind remained wide awake. She was worried that his illness was getting worse. He had never behaved this way before. The words from the caregiver's book started twirling in front of her eye, "When the full moon comes, patients become more anxious than usual and get very confused."

She herself was very disciplined. She had inherited that from her dear Dada. Sometimes she was almost a little fanatic about her routine. She was used to being home alone while he was at work, nobody to disturb her.

Now everything had changed. He was constantly perched by her side. She would have enjoyed that closeness if he had acted this way when their nest had first emptied. She began waking up a lot earlier before him to enjoy the peaceful dawns. She started taking him with her to the swimming pool; he would walk on the indoor path while she swam.

He needed to eat a healthy snack every few hours to keep his blood sugar level, so she made sure to carry food in the car and in her purse wherever they went. She could not go anywhere without first thinking of him. If she had to do any errands, he would have to be with her. It would be lunch time when they returned. So she had to plan his lunch ahead of time, so upon returning he would not start whining for food. He never took a nap. When the girls were in school, she would do Shavasan every day exactly at 3 p.m. before they came home. It would charge her battery for rest of the day. Then hot decaf coffee with a biscuit to dunk and a piece of fruit. Then time for leftover house chores, and before she knew it would be dinner time. After dinner they would go for a walk. This was their favorite ritual since they got married. But now it is a must for keeping his sugar down. She made sure not to miss it. At night after measuring his sugar, she would give him snack accordingly and get him ready for bed.

Sitting quietly at last, she would ponder, 'Where has my day gone?' She could never find the answer for this puzzle as the months passed by. The trajectory of his illness started accelerating. She accumulated more and more responsibilities of caring for him. Minor trivial work added to her routine started sucking up her strength. Weariness would conquer her as soon as she woke up, her day already mapped out in the same routines. She felt like a hamster running on the wheel continuously but getting nowhere.

After he fell asleep, all her fatigue would be awakened. She used to love to read or write her diary at bedtime. Now she was too tired for that, yet sleep would elude her. The deprivation of sleep would start a vicious cycle of more fatigue the next day.

So she found a solution to bring her own life back on track again. Yellow stickies crowded her refrigerator, grumbled when she put a long list of homework exercises for her yoga students. Even though she practiced these mental exercises often, now it will be an everyday pill.

- Dhyana-Dharana-Pranayama
- Listen to classical music.
- Social life is a must for caregivers so keep in touch and visit with friends.
- Live in the moment.
- Don't react, only respond.
- It's all in the Goddess hand, you don't have any control, so let it go.
- Think positively and act accordingly.
- My glass is always full.
- Go out of your way and make time to help others.
- Be creative in everyday life through your art, writings, etc.
- Read poetry, e.g., Rumi.
- Learn something new each day.
- Don't forget to play with Jeevan.

***

May 12, 2012

I took Madhukar for a lab test for his sodium level. He gets extremely agitated and restless when we go to any doctors, today was not an exception. His restlessness gives me a tension also, not knowing how he would react! I wrote his name on the waiting list of patients and started giving the form to the lab technician that Dr. Khera had given me, to make sure it was the right form. Dr. Khera had already sent the other necessary forms for the test directly to the lab.

But the technician said to me in an indifferent tone, "Not now, I will check it when his turn comes."

At last, after waiting a long 40 minutes, Madhukar's turn finally came. The same technician checked the paper in my hand, and without looking at me she said in a very dry voice, "This test needs fasting." I was surprised because Dr. Khera always instructs me if the text needs fasting.

"I wish you had looked at this form when I first checked in with you. It would have saved a lot of distress for my ailing husband. It makes him extremely anxious to wait like this." The words jumped out of my mouth with a little irritation. She shrugged her shoulders, avoided looking at me, and announced, "Next."

I always give praise when somebody has nice manners, whoever that might be - a salesman, nurse, waiter etc., and I pass it on to their supervisor. But today that was not going to happen; on the contrary, as soon as I came home, I reported her attitude to Dr. Khera. Next morning, I took him back again to the lab, Madhukar was upset that I did not give him breakfast. With my luck it was the same woman from the previous day. There were twelve people ahead of us. I was afraid that all the long wait, would cause his sugar to go down dangerously low, giving him hypo. My mind's eye started seeing his trembling body having a heavy sweat. I sincerely requested to the technician to take him right away to avoid his body going into shock due to his diabetes. She curtly answered, "I am the only one here, and all these people are ahead of him. I can't help you, but if you ask them, then maybe he can go ahead of them."

I was desperate, so without hesitation I helplessly announced and begged all the people in the waiting room. I explained his condition to them, and that I told them that it was not fair to them, but it would be a great favor for him. There was dead silence in the room; no one said a word, but they all nodded signaling 'yes'. Holding Madhukar's hand gently, I dashed inside to the technician. I thanked her and asked if I could get her some Dunkin coffee. She answered in a same monotonous tone, "No, I am all set."

I came back to the waiting room. I profoundly thanked and bowed to all the people again and again, I was intensely grateful for their good deed. My eyes became teary, my words heavy with gratitude, "Please let me get some coffee and donuts for all of you from Dunkin Donut's." They all shook their heads negatively, again without any words.

As soon as Madhukar came back out, I gave him his breakfast that I had brought from home and sat next to him. but I hated my vulnerable situation. My self-pity burst out forcefully, and all of my control was drowned in streaming tears. I started sobbing without any inhibitions. Madhukar looking at me with a blank face, continued shoveling his food. Poor guy - he was beyond comprehension. But I was shocked that none of the other people reached out for me. I had no right to judge or blame them. They had already fulfilled their duty by allowing Madhukar to cut in line. But the whole rest of the day I kept thinking that if I were in their place, I would not have hesitated to console a crying person… I remembered when we were at Jeevan's piano concert, there was a little girl who fell down and got a bloody knee. She started crying, and her parents were not nearby. I ran to her to wipe her tears.

I begged my goddess to give me the courage and opportunity to comfort someone's sorrow. At the same time I rebuked myself, forbidding me to be so emotional about his sickness ever again.

***

May 8, 2011

"Jyoti, *according to a famous Sanskrit shloka, an ideal wife is a manager, homemaker, lover, and secretary*, and you are like that!" Madhukar's whispers kept humming in my ears. When he was elected as the first president of our New England Marathi Mandal, I became his secretary. He gave me full freedom to plan the yearly programs which would continue in the future.

In 1980, he was a professor at UMass in Boston. While teaching there, he wrote a textbook and a guide on business management, *Management Science: A Survey of Quantitative Decision-Making Techniques.* His book became extremely popular. Of course the typist was me. Just looking at the complicated equations, my hands would start trembling. It was so difficult to write all the statistics on a typewriter, but I did it. Every time he finished a chapter, he would take us out to a nice restaurant. "I don't treat my secretary at the college like this. But you are my special and favorite secretary," he used to say.

But now it took a 360° turn; there was no trace of that favoritism anymore. He was always grumpy and angry at me. No matter how hard I tried he was never pleased with me. My name was on the blacklist. In the beginning of his illness, we would have constant arguments and quarrels, which used to make me sad. This was an unfamiliar and lonely road. Remembering my loss of his ever-smiling, talkative personality, a kernel of sadness would start gushing tears. Last two years I have become an orphan to his loving words. But unfortunately, now I become accustomed to his behavior. I tried my best to be positive in the face of his negativity and avoid any confrontation. '*Ho ho*, yes dear' became my *Mantra*. I carved his name at the top of my whitelist.

***

December 10, 2013

Her car was forced to stop again for the third time at the signal. She got irritated by the rules of the road. Since yesterday she was also hindered by red lights in her own life, which were beyond her control.

Today the same thing happened. She was going to meet her friend Dynnie after many years; it was so difficult to get their calendars to match. The caregiver who took care of Madhukar was sick and had canceled the night before. She was frustrated and disappointed, but she could not leave her husband alone now. His dementia was developing faster day by day. She was saddened to see that and felt helpless that she could not do anything. Each day, the bright ray of his brilliant personality was covered in darkness. She lost him 3 years ago, the moment the doctor had diagnosed him with Alzheimer's. She had been dedicated to him all her life but now it became her only mission. This path was not easy to walk; she was very lonely without his smile.

Finely she called Dynnie and expressed her regret for having to cancel their lunch. Dynnie told her she had to go for an MRI. "Are you ok, what's the matter?" Jyoti asked. Dynnie assured her it was not anything serious and she would still like to get together. At that very moment, her daughter Chitra entered the house. Listening to their conversation, Chitra pleaded to her mother,

"Aai, why don't you go? I will look after Daddy. You two have not seen each other for such a long time." Jyoti's eyes watered; their roles had changed, and now her daughters became her mother.

"What I would have done without you?" she murmured as she hugged Chitra. Her mind was still foggy with vulnerability. Her life was harshly controlled by the iron hands of his sickness. Today she woke up earlier than usual. Her days always started with tender loving care for him. She gave him a shower, shaved him, dressed him, and told him how handsome he looked. He was still her prince charming. Fed him his breakfast. Then brushed his teeth. She got ready for the pool. All this she had been doing for the last two years without any complaints. But she knew this phase three was going to end soon and he would no longer be able to walk on his own. She was not sure how she was going to manage him.

Chitra came to pick him up on time, with this tight rope of balancing; she finally was on her way to see Dynnie. Her favorite song was playing on the car's CD player, "Ghungatakaa pat khol," "Take off your veil. Then only will you see the hidden treasure." But before she could even try to absorb the deep meaning, her mobile shrieked. She knew it must be one of her daughters; she never gave her cell phone number to anybody else.

"Aai, did you know? One of the lenses from Daddy's eyeglasses is missing!" Chitra's words evaporated her good mood. *Oh no, now without the glasses he will be more baffled. What if somebody stepped on that delicate glass and crushed it*? The thoughts pounded in her mind. She remembered that morning while walking by the pool that he went back and forth and then stumbled as if he was looking for something. Then he took off his glasses, kept them at the edge of the pool. and lingered there for sometimes. She even scolded him gently,

"Please don't put your eyeglasses there. You will lose it."

She blamed herself for not realizing that he must have lost the lens at that time. She thought of the hawk who sat on the top of the maple tree in her back yard looking down at its prey. She could have used the hawk's sharp vision to keep an eye on her beloved husband who was the prey of this cruel disease. She described that spot to Chitra apologetically and asked her if she could go back to the pool and look for it. She knew this would add an extra burden on her daughter in her tight schedule.

The last 46 years of their married life was a big wave cradled by the full moon, but now it turned into a tsunami that they were both drowning in. She was hanging on to him by a little silk thread of her strength! 'What's the matter with me?' She became alarmed. "Live in the moment" was her motto, but today it did not come naturally to her. The wheels on the car were going forward while her mind kept slipping backwards. Bleakly she took the brakes off of her mind and allowed it to go to their enchanted past. She didn't even realize when her car came to the parking lot of the meeting place. Thankfully, the cruise control of her mind was on.

She entered Panera Bread. Dynnie was nowhere to be seen. She was also coming from a long distance, so maybe got stuck in traffic. Jyoti took a seat right next to the entrance, took her little diary from her purse and started writing the poem that was crawling out like an earthworm from her muddy mind since morning.

The clock was ticking fast. It was past 12:25 p.m. but no sign of Dynnie still. She became restless. Finally Dynnie entered. Thirty-five years ago their daughters were together in the 3rd grade and that is when they first met; their acquaintance soon sprouted into friendship.

Dynnie was tall with a net of thick, black, curly hair, a spark in her eyes, and always a little mischievous smile on her kind face. Jyoti always admired Dynnie. They used to live nearby, which made it easy to develop their closeness. They used to go for long walks. The gourmet group they belonged to was perfect for their gastronomical zeal. They were young then and lived a carefree life.

Gone are those days of wine and roses, her mind whispered. Now they were living quite far away from each other. "It has been long 3 years, where should I begin?" Dynnie gave her a big hug.

Jyoti took out the gift for Dynnie, which she carefully wrapped that morning. Inside was a print of her own painting, a beautiful young maiden "Abhisarika," one who is meeting her lover secretly on a moonlit night. Jyoti had painted it specially for Madhukar on their 10th anniversary.

Drawing and painting was her passion. Later it was thrived by his constant support like a shadow you can't separate. He was her first admirer always. Again her mind was lingering in the past. She wanted to catch those days back again, but they were like a butterfly, quick to slip away.

"Dynnie, I want to give you a part of me. This is a salute to your valuable friendship!"

"How beautiful this painting and your writing is," Dynnie read the contents behind the print and gave her another hug.

Dynnie opened the album of her recent trip photos. She was an avid and brave traveler. Her footsteps have been traced in the cold Iceland to all the way to jungles of Africa. She started describing her latest hiking in the Tibet. She had just traveled to Nepal and Tibet.

Jyoti was thrilled to witness Kailas. As the pages of Dynnie's album turned, memories unwrapped again from Jyoti's past.

"Do you like hiking?"

That was his first question to her when she met him second time before marrying him. She was puzzled! Without any trace, why in the world did he ask about mountains? Weren't there more important things about their future life together to ask about? Why in the world would he ask this silly question?

She smiled and calmly replied, "Well, I was brought up in Mumbai. So no mountains around but I have climbed 30 stairs at least 10 times every day! So you do the calculations."

He was a mathematician. After hearing her answer, a little afraid that she might not allow him to pursue his hobby, he climbed Kalsubai, the highest peak in the state of Maharashtra, just before they got married!

Later when they came to the U.S., her mountain climbing started with a little hill in their town. When their daughters were little, every fall it became a ritual to see the beautiful autumn colors on Mt. Monadnock in New Hampshire. She would be panting all the way up and suffering leg cramps, but once she reached the top, she would be so spellbound by the panorama that she would forget about all her toil and moil. The girls of course took after their father and they also raced up the mountain leaving their poor mother no alternative but to tug along, just as the tailpipe has no choice but to go along behind the car.

Once he dared her to go on the top of Mt. Washington with him. She took his challenge and even though grumbling all the way, she conquered the highest peak in New Hampshire. He had an unwritten rule, if there is a mountain nearby, he had to triumph over it. He knew all the little trails as if they were lines on his palm. She used to tease him, "You must have been a "Mawala of Mount Sahyadri" (a minuteman soldier of Raja Shivaji; together they defended all the forts against the Mughal emperor, and eventually established the free state of Maharashtra).

She started telling Dynnie her saga about the tallest peak in Great Britain, the famous Ben Nevis in Scotland. Madhukar's number one agenda during their trip was to climb it, of course. One early morning at dawn they reached the bottom of Ben Nevis. The owner of the bed and breakfast had warned them that the climb is difficult and time consuming. Madhukar had no problem with that, and she, being a *pativrata* followed him. Four hours went by with no sign of the peak. Her back started protesting, her breath started pumping, and she lost her resilience. He was not about to retreat. He was way ahead of her. The forest was so dark and deep; she did not dare to stay alone there.

Finally after eight hours she reached the top, very fatigued and unable to utter any sound. In spite of a hot summery day there was solid ice on the top of Ben Nevis. The absolute tranquility was pulling the blue sky towards her. She was intoxicated by that stillness and to her amazement her battery was completely charged within seconds. All her exhaustion completely vanished. She decided to look around. There was a little pile of rocks. By then, with all her mountaineering adventures, she knew it was a homage for climbers who had not made it. She felt heavy with that loss and went near to pay her respects. What a wonderful revelation! It was a shrine all right, not to offer condolences, but to honor the successful hikers! She was thrilled to find somebody as crazy as she was. An unknown rock lover had piled stones from the tallest mountains in the whole world. She was in seventh heaven. She started reading all the names on the rocks. There was one from Kailas and Mt. Everest! She prayed right there to Mt. Kailas, knowing that she would never be able to climb it.

'Maybe I can take that rock from Kailas,' a little greed begged but she couldn't commit such a sinful act. She dragged Madhukar to this unusual temple and they lingered there for a long time. By now the sun started drowning toward the west, and reluctantly they departed this unique place and started descending before it got too dark.

From then on, wherever she went in the world, she brought back a pebble or a small rock as a souvenir. Her rock collection had really grown. She lost her mind when they were in New Zealand; the entire beach was covered with shiny smooth gray, black and silvery rocks, and she started gathering them greedily in her sack like a child in a toy store until she saw the sign, 'PENALTY - Rocks cannot be moved from this beach'.

She had no idea how many memories had been buried under so many years of traveling. Her mundane things and taking care of her husband had masked all those wonderful memories under dark anxiety. Today after seeing Dynnie's Kailas photos, she felt a new stream of positive energy emerging.

"Dynnie, you went to Kailas, you swam in Lake Manas; it is the dream of every Indian to make this pilgrimage. I am so grateful to you for this wonderful holy Kailas Darshan. You are a lucky woman." She hugged Dynnie again and again and got up from the chair. The clock was ticking. It was getting late.

"Oh I almost forgot, here is something for you. Open it when you are home." Dynnie stuffed a gift into her hand. Jyoti reached home in a good mood, *'that's what friends do to you,'* she chuckled to herself. Chitra gave her the whole story about how she found the lens in the spot by the pool, as Jyoti had described. Evening brought all the unfinished chores since she had left early that morning. He was also waiting for her like a child. She fed him the dinner, gave him his insulin shot, and got him ready for bed. By night she was very tired, went to put the alarm at the front door and saw Dynnie's gift.

'Oh! I forgot all about it.' She opened her present in a hurry like a little girl.

Inside, there were two small rocks marked with a yellow sticky note "Mt. Kailash" and "Lake Manas." Her mind was drenched with joy, immersing again and again in the ripples of Lake Manas. She had asked everybody who had been to Manas if they had seen two white swans described in the mythic story. The reply was always 'no'.

But today by some magic those innate rocks came alive as two beautiful white swans swimming happily ever after.

***

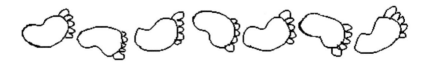

January 2012

I have to keep a constant eye on him. I have become a secret agent. He gets upset over my spying.

"Why aren't you helping me to put on my undershirt?" he growled at me.

While he was on the Namenda medication, he was able to put on his clothes most of the time, and I was purposely letting him do it himself. But then Dr. Nair stopped his prescription since the effect wears off after a few months. So now Madhukar needed my constant emotional encouragement.

"Try on your own first and if you can't do it, I will help you," I tried to coax him. "Oh, good you did it!"

While praising him I realized he had put it on inside out. I gently showed him and without any grumbling he changed it obediently. Afterwards he had fiddled around in the bathroom for a long time. Even though I was exhausted, still I had to go check if he had turned off all the lights and closed the taps. Finally, I flung my fatigued body on the bed and turned onto my left side, hoping to fall asleep. He was lying on his right-side. In reality, we had been sleeping like that mostly. But we did not turn our backs to each other intentionally. Knowing that he was next to me and listening to his steady breathing would soothe me to a beautiful mehfil of our intimacy. Today that mehfil has become silent.

I felt a huge chasm between us. We had become two mountain peaks, who could never reach to each other with a canyon between.

A love song by the famous poet Mangesh Padgaokar started resonating in my ears.

'*Bhinn dishana firat rahave natar don diwane"*
"Two lovers now roam aimlessly in opposite directions searching for each other"

Madhukar used to sing that. Who is this stranger sleeping next to me? I wanted to decode all his mute thoughts. I wished an imprint of his mind would reveal a secret message, like a bottle with a note inside washed ashore by the tides. I started choking, wanted to hold on to him, hold on to that lost hope.

"Jyoti, you really do pay attention to every minute thing while caring for me."

I pinched myself to see if this was a dream. His simple kind words startled me. I thought he was fast asleep. The goose feathers under my pillow, became alive with their silken touch. I guess stopping Namenda was a good idea. Maybe my old Raja was coming back to me. I tried to make him talk more.

"Raja, if this was the other way around, if I was sick, I know you would have taken care of me too."

"No, not at all, never. I could not take care of you the same way you do it for me," without a hesitation he confessed. I know, not everybody's nature is that of a caregiver. Still, I wanted to believe that yes, he would have taken care of me with love in spite of what he said.

A long time ago in Framingham, I had a minor surgery. The nurse was pushing me in the wheelchair to our car. She advised Madhukar, "Jyoti needs TLC today and tomorrow." He nodded to her and started driving. After reaching home, I laid down to rest. The evening shadows started spreading. Madhukar came in the room, "Jyoti what's for dinner today?" I was well aware of his absentminded nature. I got up without a word. Opened the fridge and took a casserole out for our dinner that I had made in advance.

His confession scratched the scar of another old wound. It was 1969 in Decatur. I had gone for my six-week checkup after Swati's birth. The gynecologist found a lump in my breast. He declared that he needed to do a biopsy immediately. The news shattered me. Those days, a lump in the breast would only mean cancer. I was petrified, all alone taking care of a little newborn baby. Madhukar would be at work the whole day. My day was spent in nursing, changing diapers, cleaning the house, and cooking. Not to even mention sleep deprivation. I was exhausted, moving like a zombie. Madhukar clammed up feeling stressed. In our two and half years of togetherness, I had not really accepted his way of handling stress. I tried often and in vain to help him open up.

I was restless. Who would take care of my baby? I had to stop nursing her immediately in order to dry out the milk in the breast. The pain was stabbing. Nobody had heard of breast pumps. I had to go buy bottles, formula, a sterilization - all a new untimely adventure. What if I did not survive? What would happen to my baby? The hornet's nest opened to release a thousand stinging questions and doubts.

My friend Sue Zimmerman from our apartment complex became my angel. She offered to take care of Swati. She was a nurse, and her own son was about a year old. Her kindness as an experienced mom gave me a slight relief. I did not want to scare Aai Dada, so I could not ask for their advice. The future kept mocking me all night while I waited the morning of the biopsy procedure. They were pushing me on the gurney to the operating room. Madhukar was walking next to me. I clasped my hand in his tightly, kept telling him again and again, "I want you to be by my side when I hear the biopsy results. Please be there with me."

"Ok," I barely could hear through his quivering lips, his fearful eyes staring at me like a lamb going to slaughter. When I became conscious again, I kept looking for him. But I was all alone in the room. Just then the doctor walked in and smiled at me,

"Mrs. Joshi, not to worry, the result came, it's benign!"

I was extremely relived by his assurance but realizing that my mate was not by my side swept all the joy away; his absence pierced the oozing wound for a long time. When he returned after a few hours, I asked him furiously,

"Where were you? I told you to be by my side when I wake up!"

"Oh, I asked the doctor, when you would wake up. He could not tell me an exact time. He told me that he had gotten the results right away from the lab and everything was fine. Not to worry. I was relieved to hear that. I found out at the last minute that there was an important meeting at the office. He told me to go ahead," he calmly tried to justify his absence.

He was absent minded, I knew him, he did not do that purposely, but I was extremely disappointed. I realized his job would always have priority over his wife. He used to get so absorbed in his work that sometimes he would forget to eat his lunch. When I would open his lunchbox, I would find food that was untouched, or half eaten. How could I compete with his quest for his sincere, hard work?

Over the years, it still kept happening. If I ever got sick, he would bombard me with all kinds of medicines, but not a single word of compassion. I used to get upset but understood he is like a coconut, with a hard shell to crack but with sweet creamy tender meat inside. He could never truly be able to unload his feelings.

I wonder if it came from his childhood. He was always shifted from one aunt to another or sometimes from his grandparents' home to his parents, back and forth because his father was unable to support his family. His father had been busy in the fight for independence and had never gotten the education required for a steady job. Maybe Madhukar never experienced a comforting loving pat on his back or any kind words from his relatives. So how would a young child learn compassion? For that he needed coaching from my Dada. I think later whenever Dada came to visit us, Madhukar observed and learned from Dada's compassionate nature.

Today after a long time, I had found my long-lost Raja. I turned towards him, even though he was asleep, I patted lovingly on his back whispering, "I love you unconditionally, so sleep soundly, my sweetheart!"

He snapped back at me, "It's not true at all, you are trying to bribe me".

His sharp words cut me through and through, wiping away my loving pledge. I forgot his sickness, lost my endurance, and fired at him, "No matter how much I try hard, you just don't see anything good in me anymore! I am going to move in with Chitra. You can do whatever you feel like. You will have to take care of yourself," the words kept shooting out too fast to swallow them.

***

Next morning I was heading to the pool. My car was at the traffic light. I always love to gaze at the weeds of the divider island on the road. Wildflowers amidst them swinging on a breeze, drew me in, to forget my stress. I rolled down the window to hear their whispers:

Every morning without a miss
we see her in her blue Corolla.
waiting eagerly at the red light
as if she stopped there just to observe us.
She opens the car window to salute us,
her curly black locks gently swinging with the breeze.
Our pink color readily blends into her smile.
She looks deep into our hearts.
Her admiration assures us that our day is going to be a grand success.
The empty cigarette packages,
dry, worn out French fries,
old haggard plastic grocery bags,
poisonous black smoke from the cars,
and overgrown wild grass goes without any notice just for a second.
Just for a second!
Our buds ready impatiently to bloom with her smile.
We find new hope to live,
even in the midst of the roaring giant lawnmower rushing toward us.
We kept blooming just for her.

The shrieking horn of the car behind me crumbled my magical moment. I turned my car towards the pool. Hoping the waves in the pool were waiting for me like those wildflowers. I entered the warm water and started my usual water-aerobics workout, but my threat to Madhukar from last night boomeranged towards me, slowing me down. The bubbles of remorse started bursting, and the tsunami of guilt drowned me. My own cruelty towards him paralyzed me. I begged the water to caress me and began confessing.

It was just a mere vacant threat, nothing else.
Poor thing, it's not his fault, he is not to be blamed.

The real culprit is that merciless disease.
I will not be burned in his fury but will rise like a phoenix.
I will borrow Sita's Agnidivya and reappear as a peaceful glow.
Dreams of hope will grow in my womb.
I will retreat into the forest of his happy memories.
I will wait for eternity to hear the flute of his soul.
Just one melody.
Just one tune.
Only from you, my Raja.
Only from you.

***

November 5, 2013

After dinner we went out for our evening stroll. I held his hand to give him support. The autumn sky was covered with a pitch-dark blanket. I signaled Madhukar to look up in the sky, "Look at that lovely bright star Venus." Somehow, my Raja's dim light twinkled. Just like in the old days, he corrected me immediately, "Jyoti, it's not a star. It's a planet." I was stunned listening to his words. He called my name, and he seemed normal for a split second. My mind started humming an old Marathi song in which Venus was called a star.

Shukra tara mand wara, chandane panyatuni, chandra ahe, swapn vahe dhund ya ganyatuni.
Venus the evening star, soft breeze, moonlight reflected on the water, a dream flows through in this captivating moment.

This used to be our normal dialog; he would correct me about some astronomy fact.

I lingered in that enchanted melody, but in the next flash Venus disappeared behind the clouds, just like Madhukar has become foggy to me. Now he really doesn't recognize who I am anymore. '*It's ok, you recognize him! Then it's all right, he is still your old Raja. He will be always close to you.*' My weepy mind tried to reassure me.

Like all the others in those days ours was a proposed marriage. Our parents introduced us initially. We never dated each other. So many days and months after our wedding were spent in trying to know each other, and it is still continuing. After 46 year of togetherness, I was beginning to understand him in a totally different new way, as if I had just met him.

My memories started sparkling. All four of us crammed lovingly on the sofa, watching the news after dinner. They announced that after thousands of years, a rare phenomenon was going to occur. Saturn, Mars, and Jupiter would appear to be in a straight line. I knew my husband was definitely going to be awake at 2 a.m. to observe this.

"Me too!" 8-year-old Chitra insisted on watching it with her Daddy. So both of them went to bed early with the alarm set for 1:45.

As soon as we were married Madhukar started teaching me the planets and stars on our daily walks. Watching the solar system and constellations was Madhukar's passionate hobby. He would always point to Venus in the night sky. I would crane my neck and just say, "Yes I see it," not really interested in the solar system. I was a newlywed bride, tickled that my husband was so romantic, showing me *Shukra Tara*.

When we were on the cruise for our 25th anniversary, Madhukar would be on the top deck of the ship every night observing the solar system. Before you know it, he started teaching the other passengers about astronomy. He would read every book on astronomy he could get his hands on. He would have thick texts books on the planets as bedtime reading. Later our daughters surprised their Daddy on his 60th birthday with a big 5-foot-tall telescope. He and our next-door neighbor Larry would carry that telescope into the cul de sac and gazing at the stars for hours ... at least that's what they used to tell me.

I used to warn them, "Be aware if you get caught peeping, Saturn might turn his *Vakri-drushti*[29] on you!" I must admit that I was indeed

---

[29] Vakri drushti- In Hindu astrology, planets of the Solar System other than the Sun and the Moon that appear to move backwards, which apparent motion is due to earth's orbit. Vakri in Sanskrit means twisted or crooked; so in this content it means that Saturn would curse.

thrilled to see the rings around Saturn the first time through that telescope. That telescope really heightened his passion for his hobby. He even joined the astronomy club at Wheaton College when we moved to Norton.

In 2002, when we were at our 'Windsong' home in Nashua, NH, we had a great opportunity to watch a meteor show. I was genuinely enjoying gazing at the stars, especially as I was in Madhukar's company. Night began to fall, I put two chairs on the back deck, brought two mugs of hazelnut-flavored coffee, and we sat together under the warm quilt. It was a pin-drop silence. Then one by one the stars began shooting. Supreme firework started bursting in a spectacular show. I had never seen anything like that before, making me speechless before the creator. Was it Shiva's dance?

***

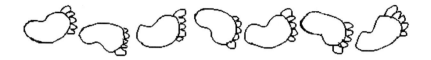

Bite huye din yaad aah gaye. Memories brought back long last days. - from the Hindi film First Love

2012

The song tumbled from my lips. What was the use of remembering old memories now? One can never catch the sunshine at night. Madhukar's behavior was like that of a light bulb. Sometimes a flicker, sometimes very dim, and suddenly it will be brightly shining. I never knew what to expect from him. As if when his brain connection was shaky then he wouldn't say anything or do anything normally. But I kept talking to him constantly as if everything were normal. "Tomorrow there is a block party, would you like to go?"

"Yes, yes! I like to meet people." His answer gave me 100 watts of power. But at the same time his normalcy would disrupt my peace of mind, making me doubt if his Alzheimer's was real? Maybe he was misdiagnosed by the doctors. Hope would start dancing like a firefly in the darkness of my mind. Yesterday I was a little late to tie his shoes. He roared like an angry lion, "When I call you, Jyoti, you must stop what you are doing and immediately come to my service! Otherwise I would not consider you to be an obedient wife."

I was stunned to hear that from him, not an attitude he ever had before. The same firefly flicker ignited wildfire in my mind. Sometimes he can't see the things that are right before his eyes. My instructions wouldn't make it past the eye-ear-brain connection. I had to physically hand it to him. But when I kept his favorite dark chocolate on the kitchen counter to see his reaction, as soon as he was near there, he snatched it and gobbled it like a hungry animal.

As night approached, I got him ready for bed. I was really tired, eager to go to sleep. But as usual he started probing me,

"Did you close the front door and turn the alarm on? Did you put my sugar measurement chart near my bed? Where is my machine?"

I tried to stay calm and answered, "It is on your dresser. I already measured your sugar tonight. Why do you ask?"

"Oh I just wanted to test you. See if you knew where it was."

"Did I do well in the test?" I quizzed him back. But he was already sound asleep.

Last week I had just returned from the book club meeting. Usually he would get mad at me for leaving him alone at home even though Chitra was with him, just like Swati used to be angry when I left her with a sitter. I was preparing myself for his artillery fire of angry words. So I asked him softly,

"Raja would you like some coffee?"

Instantly in a loving tone he said, "Jyoti, while you were away, I realized one thing. You are extremely romantic but at the same time you are very practical. You really take good care of me."

My mind so desperately wanted to shackle this newly found old Madhukar. I remembered reading that highly intelligent people, especially mathematicians, become victims of this illness. Because of their brightness, these patients managed to hide the dementia or keep it under control. When his or her disease advances, it becomes a waterfall with a strong force that no rock can survive under it.

My daughters and I always wondered how he was still able to work? How did he manage? How come his colleagues didn't see or question his behavior? Or was he the old Madhukar in the office where he has to be on his guard? Like a mother tries to find some excuse for her child misbehaving, I would find some meek justification for his strange behavior. But I knew that pretty soon I would run out of those excuses. His syndrome was just going to get stronger. What could I do to defeat it? I would try to balance on the knife edge of my worries helplessly.

***

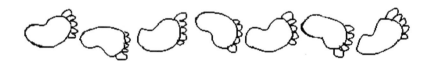

Music is a higher revelation than all wisdom and philosophy. Music is the electrical soil in which the spirit lives, thinks and invents. – Ludwig van Beethoven

June 2012

'Lagi re sawariya tuse aakhiya, Sohani sundar surat...
My eyes only see you my beloved, your lovely face'.

Kalapini's sweet melodies are so touching. Jyoti had only seen her before on YouTube. Now this goddess of harmony was sitting in front of her. Her turmeric-colored sari with a sap green blouse added more magic to her golden skin. A big red Kumkum on her forehead. A silk black thread necklace holding a copper amulet that was probably given by her guru and father, Pandit Kumar Gandharv. All her talent in the vocal arts glowing on her face. A tattered notebook in front of her contained all the *Bandishe* passed down to her from her guru. She started singing a *Nirguni* Bhajan.

'*Dusareke sang nahi jaungi, guruji mai to ek Niranjan laungi*'…I will not go with anybody else. My guru, you are the only one. I will only light one Diya. I don't need other light.

After many months she was attending a classical mehfil in Boston. The superhighway's Chakravyuh couldn't panic her; she skillfully triumphed over that labyrinth like an expert charioteer. If on that long-ago day, Madhukar had not pushed her from the Hilton's comfortable room, she would have never reached here today.

April 1969 – Chicago

They were married just six months ago, the honeymoon still lingering. Madhukar had to attend a business meeting and she had come along. Chicago's hustle and bustle reminded her of her cherished Bombay. She felt so alive. Their hotel was on Michigan Avenue, and to her delight Chicago's famous Art Institute - her Mecca - was just down the road. She spent the entire day admiring the art in the institute. Next day morning he asked her, "So where is *Rani Sarkar*- the Queen's round today?"

"Raja, why would I need to go anywhere when my Pandhari is just around the corner?"

"No, not there again, you must visit the science museum today. They have a coal mine in the dungeon. It's a unique experience. You must," Raja turned into a dictator.

She had only left Bharat few months ago and was still clutching so hard to all the memories so close to her heart. The strands of her happy childhood days pulled at her as if she were a Kathputali, a marionette. Early dawn without miss, her mother would warm the water for their baths on the coal stove. Every week the servant Bhaiya delivered a sack of coal to their doorstep from the depot. Nobody could see his real face because he would be covered head to toe in soot.

"Coal mine? What is there to see? I don't like to go into dungeons. Besides, I don't even know how to go there." Her disagreement was definitely not subtle.

"You are not a timid girl. I will show you the map. You have a car at your fingertips. You can drive there easily. You have to go," he kept on insisting.

As soon as she got her license, she started driving. She owed that to him. He had taught her real driving. She had learned firsthand how hard it was having her husband as her driving instructor. The strings of the tanpura started beating to the memories of that particular Sunday morning when he had said,

"Let's go for a ride. You drive. I want to see what Mr. Johnson is teaching you."

She proudly sat behind the steering wheel and started the car. But somehow that day the car was acting very funny; it would not go where she wanted.

"From tomorrow, no more of your Indian cultural lessons to Mr. Johnson. The devil must have a dual control brake under his foot, giving you impression that you are driving properly. His driving lessons must stop. I will teach you from now on."

She was sad and disappointed. She really liked Mr. Johnson's curious nature. He was so interested in Indian culture. There was nobody else to talk to during the day, and she was enjoying his company, happy to tell him all about her life in India. Next month the wheels kept running side by side, listening to the arguments churning between him and her. She told him that if somebody else was there instead of her, she would have divorced Madhukar instantly. She would not recommend to any of her Indian friends to learn driving from their husbands.

The day arrived for her driving test. She became nervous about the whole process. According to Madhukar, with her luck she got the softy examiner who was more interested in her sari. She was the only 'exotic' Indian woman in the town. Eyeing her beautiful jewelry, he asked if she was a princess from India. And in all that inquest, he forgot to give her a parallel parking test. She got her license. As she was driving back home, her sweet childhood started racing with her car. Yes, she was indeed a princess, pampered by her Dada. She had never known how meagre his salary actually was.

Now the car keys were hooked on her finger permanently. She was a free bird. Sometimes she would even become a backseat driver, forgetting that Madhukar was the one who had taught her!
"Let me show you the map." A gentle tap on her shoulder brought her back to the present.

She was still not used to following the map while driving at the same time. Not to mention, she could never refold the map properly according to him. The thought of reading the signs above and at the same time keeping her eyes on the road worried her. She was intimidated by the maze of superhighways in Chicago. The traffic was rough comparing to Decatur. She still didn't dare to go out of town on her own. Her youth jammed in her mind again. Her college was about to start.

"From tomorrow on, you have to take a local train from Dadar to Victoria Terminus."

She was petrified when her elder brother Aba ordered her. She had never gone on her own to the Fort area, the chaotic hub of Bombay. Never mind taking the train alone to that busy area, she was uncomfortable even taking a bus to college.

Madhukar was nagging her now, "Jyoti, you have to go, you must try."

She bit her lip concluding that all the men are just heartless. Was he the same man who had whispered in her ears last night with all that sugar-coated romantic poetry?

Frustration started streaming from her eyes. She sobbed, "How can you be so cruel? How can I go all by myself to such a long distance?"

In the end, she gave in and submissively strapped herself into the seatbelt as she started the car. Once she was on the highway, she realized she could easily pass the other cars. Before she knew it, she had parked her car in a parallel parking spot at the science museum. She couldn't get over how interesting the coal mine was. It was not gloomy as she had expected. She really enjoyed the whole experience as if she had discovered a diamond in the mine. She tasted the same wanderlust as from her college days. Back then she would walk endlessly in the Fort area after classes ended, feeling exuberant about her newly found freedom.

On the way back to the hotel, she was gliding on the six lanes of the superhighway. No stress at all - it was a piece of cake. She abruptly swerved towards an exit after seeing a billboard for an Indian grocery store. Decatur did not have such a luxury. Madhukar had to take her fifty miles away for her monthly supply of dal and mung beans. She started putting all kinds of lentils, spices, fresh coriander, barfi, canned Gulab jamun, and whatnot into her cart, like a little girl in a doll store. The store was owned by a Sardarji, who was amazed to hear this country girl's adventure in the big city. He offered her sweet mango lassi as his way of showing appreciation to this new desi sister. No more inhibition about superhighways. She had found a flying chariot. In the evening she tooted her own horn, "Raja, I must confess. You were right. It was a very unusual and exciting visit to the coal mine. Thank you for opening that magical door of confidence for me."

In 1985 they were in Ayr, Scotland for his work. There he had the opposite order, forbidding her to drive anywhere since the rental car was registered by his company in his name only. In that regard he could have competed with her Dada, who would never allowed Jyoti to ride with him in his office car to her college, which was next door to his office. Madhukar would never use the company phone to make long-distance calls or take any office supplies for his personal use.

Not only had Jyoti conquered all the territory around Ayr by foot, but she took a train by herself 100 miles away to Glasgow's famous art museum. It was the last day in Ayr. She was bored of sitting in the hotel room. He was at work. The car was just sitting idly in the hotel parking lot. Her rebellious nature peeped, and she could not resist. In the evening when he returned, she guiltily confessed, "I took a ride to a hill where beautiful homes of Ayr sat overlooking to the ocean. But I brought the car safely back!"

In the whirlpool of memories, his absence started drowning her. She longed for him now more than ever. She realized that the harsh sentence of this Alzheimer's was not only for him but her also. She felt torn and selfish to leave him at home and attend the mehfil all by herself. They always went together to listen to Indian classical music concerts. Their union was a mehfil itself, a harmonious melody of joy and love. But now the strings of the tanpura were broken. He had had a beautiful voice. When this disease started creeping silently in, and he would just sit there with his vacant eyes staring at the ceiling, she used to beg him,

"Raja, why don't you sing? Maybe you can practice a little."

"Jyoti, my voice can't utter! She knew that he couldn't think of the words. Sound is lost, melody is no more. This is the bitter truth!"

Kalapini's allap pleaded in her mind:

Did you forget, my beloved?
My words are yours too; we speak the same language.
We never had that separating line between us.
There was never even a shadow between us.
The sound that bellows from your lungs is mine.
I am your Gandhari.
All I want to see is your neck swaying to the beat.
That will last me for a lifetime.

Ganga na jaungi, Jamuna na jaungi,
na koi Teertha nahungi, dusreke sath nahi jaungi.
Nahi jaungi, nahi jaungi, nahi jaungi
I won't go to the holy Ganga, nor to the Jamuna River.

I don't need any holy water to purify me.
I will not go with anybody except you.
I won't go, I won't go, I won't go.

Kalapini's bhajan filled the entire hall. Jyoti's mind began to sing side by side with Kalapini.
Lagi re sawariya tuse aakhiya …

My eyes only see you, my beloved.
My beloved, I am all ears,
listening to Kalapini's raga Multani.
Only for you, only for you.
You are sitting next to me so close.
I am holding you within the caves of my heart.
How can we be separated?
You are flowing through my veins.
You are resonating in my heartbeat.

***

October 11, 2012

The sunrays peeping through the drape's gap warmed my face. My eyes squinted just a little. You were still snoring next to me. For a magical moment, I thought the *Jeevan Chakra*, wheel of life, was spinning smoothly but the shrieking alarm of the clock jolted me back to cruel reality.

I guide you into the shower and hand a bar of lavender soap to you, signaling to you to use it as if it is going to wash away your malady.
I dab the towel gently on your body, hoping with some magic, the towel might wipe my tears too.
I give you a clean-cut shave, but in the dark forest of my mind, bristly stubs of horrid thoughts grow uncontrollably.
The sprinkle of Old Spice on your cheeks makes my suffering more pungent.
I carry on as if everything is normal… What is normal after all?
I set the breakfast table, put the CD on, 'Open the veil, then only you can see your beloved.'
Like sunshine underneath the cloudy sky my smile shines back for a moment.
I start swimming in the pool and the waves cuddle me.
You are doing endless rounds on the edge of the pool trying to find yourself,
only to get lost and more confused.
A splinter of despair keeps getting stuck in my heart.
You come back to your chair on the deck to check that your red jacket is still dangling.
I keep it there so you will recognize your usual spot.
But the color of your red jacket signals the danger ahead.
I can't make a simple stop to do an errand.
You need to go to pee.
You get restless.
I come home and then you bug me for lunch even though you just had a banana and yogurt for snack.
Still I feed you a full lunch, and like an infant you start dozing off right at the table.
I feel pity on you.
The cobweb of your thoughts must be terrifying.
The splinter in my heart is still throbbing.

I take you to the bathroom and do the same routine.
Make sure you are secured on the sofa and help you to lie down.
Then only I climb upstairs.
Downstairs walls begin to echo with your snoring.
Ah! It must be nap time.
'Everything is normal after all', I assure myself and turn the computer on.
I need to send an important email to the insurance company.
A splinter in my heart is still prickly but now I feel a thick layer is covering my skin.
It must be the new normal!

***

January 17, 2013

Vermilion burst all over in the east. She was awake at the crack of dawn but had no energy to get up. In the past, her morning would progress in a smooth pace, as she would start doing her yoga postures, Pranayama and Dhyana. Now the clock was provoking and controlling her daily routine. She dismissed the temptation to stay in bed and abandoned the warmth of the goose down quilt. Nowadays a good night's sleep had become rare as a unicorn. No matter what, she would awake in the middle of the night. The thoughts of what lies ahead would poke at her, confiscating the rest of her sleep. When everything was normal, not even once had she thought about the future. She was living her life fully. She stared at his sleeping figure, so peaceful, not a single trace of illness on his face. The list of her things to do started crowding in her fatigued brain. Whatever chores he could do in the past had been forced on her now. Same way his confusion has oppressed him. 'I need to order his meds today, it would take an hour easily,' she murmured to herself. The calendar on the wall fluttered, reminding her of his eye appointment. Ever since he had cataract surgery, he thinks the doctor is going to operate on him again. No matter how much she tried to convince him otherwise, he would get very worked up when they went there. Next week is his dentist. Constant appointments. The doctors are never on time and waiting endlessly in that environment makes him very fidgety, going back and forth to the bathroom. She feels very awkward to enter the restroom with him.

"Good Morning!"

"Utha ho sakala jana, wache smarawa gajanana. It's time to wake up and sing the lord Ganpati's praise," she tries so hard to be cheerful.

She prepared the needle to measure his sugar. His endocrinologist had warned her that she would have to keep an eye on his sugar level from now on since he was no longer capable of that. The nurse instructed her on how to give him a shot of insulin and told her to practice on an orange the first few times. Her stomach cringed when she had to poke him with that sharp needle the first time. Luckily, the next day her cousin Kalyani and her husband Dr. Suresh came for a visit. She felt a little relieved giving Madhukar insulin under Suresh's guidance for the next two days. She chuckled to herself, how relative everything is; after only a week of practice, it was a piece of cake for her. Dada had wanted so much for his daughter to become a doctor. This is as far as she had come to the medical field.

Madhukar started getting sick often in the past few years with minor illnesses. His Alzheimer must have already set in, with hindsight she realizes. The first summer after moving to Norton they had rented a house on the beach at Cape Cod. The whole family was together. She had to be on guard holding his hand because he started losing his balance once in a while around that time. He wanted to ride his bike, despite her begging him not to. The inevitable happened; he fell down from the bike and broke his shoulder. So again there were endless visits to the doctors, to the lab for x-rays, followed by twice a week trips for physical therapy. She felt as if her own strength had been fractured. He became furious when his bike was hidden away.

Later, on every trip they took, he started getting sick. In China he had whooping cough. When they were in Prague, he cut himself while shaving, didn't realize it and kept going over and over the cut with his shaver. The cut got severely infected, and she had to take him to the hospital in a foreign country. The language barrier made it so difficult to get him right treatment immediately. As their plane was landing back in Massachusetts, his ear drum got ruptured and she had to take him directly to the ear and throat specialist. After examining Madhukar's ear, the doctor told her that he would have to do surgery on it, with the grim consequence that he might have to cut the ear. When the doctor found out about his Alzheimer's diagnosis, he was doubtful about Madhukar's capacity to go through such a serious surgery. A long month to wait and anticipate the gruesome future ahead. But a miracle happened. Just a day before his surgery, when she took him for pre-op testing, the doctor announced that by sheer luck his ear was healed.

She takes him to the sink; he keeps washing his hands continuously, turning into Lady Macbeth. Then he keeps rinsing his mouth unendingly, while the tap water is flowing in full force. She gets annoyed at such a waste of water. "*Babano*, conserve *the water*," her Aai's constant pleading.

All the memories start flowing like water through the gaps between her fingers. In Narayan Niwas, the water pressure was so low that it would not pump all the way to the third floor where they lived. The landlord was not going to do anything about it due to a lack of money. So all the males - Dada, Baba, mama, kaka, brothers in the house would form an assembly line on each floor, passing buckets full of water until her Aai was sure the 4 feet drum was full. Their entire family of ten people would have to repeat the same chore the next day. So she has been practicing her Aai's advice ever since. But now she will have to ignore his sin of wasting water. "It's time for a shower," she steered him. To make him stand stably in the shower is a tussle. She gets all wet while trying to get him to stand and suddenly he loses his balance. Her hands slippery from soap, she struggles to keep her own balance, clutching on to him. *I don't know how long I can do this.* All her confidence washes down the drain.

She manages to bring him out of the shower stall and helps him to sit on a chair. She wipes his body with an extra soft towel. His podiatrist had told her to check his feet, in between the toes, extra carefully. Then rubs the special cream he had given her. Diabetes can cause skin problems. She realizes that the tube is almost empty. She will have to renew the prescription. It will be too long to wait for another month, when his three months appointment is scheduled. Now she gets busy putting his attire on. Finally the belt is on, and last goes the hearing aids. She quickly notes in her mind to make an appointment with the audiologist also. She starts combing his hair.

She wipes his glasses clean and puts them on him; he can't even do such a simple thing on his own anymore. The brain can't estimate the distance. The same thing happens when he goes to sit on a chair, and inevitably he misses it. Morning has only begun, but her energy has merged into twilight. "Now my groom is ready," she teases. Even though she is not sure how he will react she tries to add a little humor to keep her own sanity intact.

"Here, you should drink this whole glass," she hands him his pills. He doesn't drink water at all nowadays. At the breakfast table after securing him on the chair, she starts feeding him, with extra TLC. Suddenly he barks at her,

"Where are my medicine pills? Did you take the banana? Help me to put on my jacket!"

Short term memory forces him to forget what he did a minute ago. She swallows her pride and controls her tears. When Kalyani and Suresh were here, he was screaming at her in the same manner, and she had felt very humiliated. "Did you see how he treats me?" she asked Suresh through her sobs.

"Jyoti, he does not have anyone but you. He knows how much you love him. You are his only companion. Who else could he lash out at but you?"

Even though she knew this, listening to Suresh's wisdom she fell apart. Now after much practice she has embraced that understanding. She has learned to evaporate her tears. It's time to go, she muffles and puts her winter jacket on after she has done his first. Immediately he announces that he needs to go to the bathroom. She knows it's just mania, not a true urge, but she can't take any chances. So from A to Z, the whole circus act begins again. Take the jacket off, remove the belt, take the pants off again and on again!

I want my freedom back. Her mind revolts. She has hired caretakers for him, but she has to dance to their timetable. She has to juggle between the insurance company, his doctor's visits, his meds. All the negative thoughts swarm like mosquitoes in the swamp. Outrage suffocates her. *Why does he have to latch on to me constantly? His closeness is strangling me.* The thought snaps at her like a gusty wind violently shuts the door. She is alarmed by her attitude. She feels like a proper stranger to herself. She becomes ashamed by her selfishness. How can I even think like that? The guilt has muddied her completely. With him sitting next to her, she drives like an android.

At the pool she immerses, starts swimming wildly. Slowly the warm water calms her. As if the holy Ganga has mixed in the pool water, all her negativity melts away and she finds her true self. All the love, commitment and devotion for her Raja comes back, overlapping her. At last she is at peace.

***

That same afternoon Kathleen came for tea, a visit that was long overdue. She was Jeevan's swim teacher at the pool and was aware of Madhukar's condition. She had seen his nonstop rounds around the pool, checking constantly for his red jacket. I had told his situation to all the workers there just in case he ever left the premises. I wasn't able to keep eye on him while I was in the changing room.

But when Kathleen entered the house, Madhukar started acting very strangely…hiding behind me as soon as he saw her. He pulled my hand abruptly. I think he did not like that I was chatting with her. I remembered when Chitra was a toddler she would do the same thing when my friends came for a visit. He became a toddler who didn't want to share his mother with Kathleen. Watching his behavior, Kathleen said,

"Jyoti, now that he's controlling your life like this, do you resent him? You have no freedom left. You must hate him."

"No, never! I love him so much. He is ill. He never controlled me before. His Alzheimer's is controlling him and that is why he acts like that, Kathleen. Our love is not so weak that I will ever abandon him or hate him." Sharp words shot from the quiver of my mind.

It was only a little after 3:30 p.m. when Kathleen left. Madhukar began pacing back and forth. He went to the living room and abruptly he stalled near the window. I thought he was looking out at the pink rays of sunset. But suddenly he pulled the shades down and zipped the curtain. Then he continued to pull the window curtains closed all over the house. The untimely darkness made me depressed, choking like a monster. *'Why are you shutting the curtains? The sunlight is so limited in the winter',* luckily in time my lips also zipped the words shut and my mind drew the curtains of compromise. I figured that perhaps his own reflection in the window must have confused him and made him think that there was a stranger staring at him. I tried mightily to stay calm but at the same time all the worries of future put a heavy weight on my back. My strength started fading away with the vanishing sun on the horizon.

I couldn't carry this weight of his care all by myself anymore. When I came to America, I had learned to be self-dependent out of necessity. When I started working full-time as well as giving yoga classes in the evening, I decided to hire outside help. Every two weeks Siddha, a young Brazilian woman, came to clean the house. To give her all that money for just two hours was unbearable for me. But Madhukar insisted that we continue with Siddha so that I could have some of my own time back. It didn't take long for Siddha with her kind nature to become a part of our family, just like Kashi our maid was in Dadar while I was growing up. Siddha stayed with us until we left Framingham.

'Nobody would take care of him like me, with love and affinity,' was my firm belief. But my constant struggle with bodily exhaustion convinced me to look for outside help. It was not as easy a task as I had expected. After long hours of many phone calls and interviews, I chose a company with male caregivers. I thought Madhukar would be more at ease while taking a shower and get dressed under John's supervision. On the contrary, he became infuriated and refused to co-operate with John. Next day I was back to my duty.

I next hired the VNA company after recommendation from my neighbor. The caregivers were all females. I decided to try them for two hours every other day. I spent a lot of time explaining Madhukar's needs to the first woman upon her arrival. Two hours went by too fast. I was not happy when the next time a different woman appeared at the house. Again I had to go through my instructions. Madhukar would get extremely uncomfortable adjusting to a different person every time. I did not like the inconsistency either. They were not taking care of him with dignity and affection. They were never on time, would always have many excuses, and leave five to ten minutes early. It became an extra balancing act for me that I didn't need. So I had to look for another company. The same pattern kept repeating. I was ready to pull my hair out in desperation. After changing agencies for a year, I finally found a wonderful company, Visiting Angels. Truly, all the caregivers were angels. They assigned only two women on weekdays and one on weekends. By then Madhukar had really declined rapidly. Not only his abilities to function were demolished but his cognitive skills were gone. He no longer complained or protested while they gave him a shower or changed his diapers. Silvia came two hours in the morning. She would take pride in dressing him as if he were going to the office. He obediently followed her like a good boy. Ellie was younger than Chitra and built like her. I think may be that Madhukar often thought she was Chitra. Even though she addressed him as Dr. J, it was said so lovingly as if she were indeed his daughter.

She would come in the evening, take him for a walk, and get him ready for bed. If my flower vase were empty, Ellie would bring flowers from the back yard. Silvia would bring fresh figs for Madhukar, once she found that he liked them. Mary would come on weekends and read to Madhukar or play games with him, not in the least bothered by his impassiveness. They were all extremely gentle and knew how to take care of his special needs. Talking softly to him always. They were not just doing their job as caregivers but poured their heart into it. Madhukar had also became a gentle soul now as the nurse Joyce had been forecasting. I was beginning to relax and was able to find some time for myself. With their loving gesture it didn't take long before the Visiting Angels became our family members. Mary was very much interested to learn how to meditate so I happily taught her. I was extremely grateful to these three angels.

One day Silvia was sick, so a different care giver Monica showed up, actually a little earlier than the usual time. She seemed very old for this kind of job. I was concerned about how Madhukar would react to this proper stranger. I took her to the bedroom where Madhukar was still sleeping.

"Have you worked with Alzheimer's patients?" looking at her wrinkled face I anxiously asked her. "I volunteer with autistic children," she smiled at me.

Then she took her shoes off without my asking, and immediately took charge of Madhukar as if she had been coming to us every day. This was a pleasant surprise; I didn't have to go through any instructions. I noticed that she was wearing a locket with an angel in it.

"Did you know I collect angels?" I said to her.

"Where is your collection?" she asked while curiously looking around.

"You will find them all over the house, some of them are hiding. There is a special angel in here today," I said, staring at her meaningfully as I showed her around the house.

***

Christmas, December 2011

My very first Christmas party was at Madhukar's boss Dr. Eicker in1967 in Decatur. While growing up in Dadar, surrounded by a mostly Hindu community I was never exposed to Christian celebrations. The idea of bringing a pine tree inside the house and decorating it with twinkling lights brightened my mind tremendously in that snowy wintery Midwest weather. So that tradition began in the Joshi house, even before our two daughters were born. When Swati and Chitra were little, I was always trying very hard to introduce them all the Indian celebrations and cultural traditions. It was a balancing act, and not easy because of the vast difference between the outside world and inside the house like the North and South poles. Later when they were in college, Indian culture and Marathi language started fading away a little bit. Observing their youth, full of zest I loosened the strings of my apron.

Now as an adult my darling girls have become my dear friends. Since Jeevan's birth we started celebrating Christmas at Chitra's house. Today was the same. Swati had come early to help me with Madhukar. It was late at night as we returned home after getting stuffed with the delicious Christmas feast. I was very tired and eager to put my head on the pillow. I pulled back the covers and saw an envelope. I knew right away that it must be from Swati. It brought smile to me, as I started reading it eagerly…The picture on the card stunned me. A little girl was stuck in a chasm between two mountains. In front of her there was a pillar that was ready to fall on her. It was so huge she would be crushed instantly. So she was trying with all her might to push it away. A picture speaks a thousand words. The card gave me an instant megadose of courage.

'Dear Aai, I know you are carrying a heavy burden on your shoulders. But please remember, you are not alone. We are all with you. I will come every weekend and sleep over on alternate weekends. You are taking such good care of Daddy. He is lucky to have you. Aai, I love you so much. I will call you every day, so you won't be lonely. Lots of xxxooo, Swati'.

Swati's heartwarming, tear-jerking words made me speechless. So, so grateful to my Devi for giving me Swatu and Chitru. Every time Madhukar showered me with a gift of precious gems, I used to tell him, "Why do you have to buy me these? I am the mother of two beautiful jewels, my shiny *nakshatra*, my sweet *chimanya*-little sparrows." After he became ill, I showed them how to give him a shot of insulin. Now he had become their *chimana bal*- baby bird. They both came regularly to help me to feed him, give him baths, and dress him. Without their solid loving support I would not have been able to take care of him. I was fully aware of their commitment and will always be indebted to them. Not every shiny stone is a diamond until it is tested. They passed this difficult test with flying colors and became my invaluable gems. I have often expressed my gratitude to them. They had tied us around their pinkies always by their loving nature.

I recalled that January when Chitra was in 6th grade. She didn't have a house key since I was always home by the time the girls would return from school. It was our anniversary. I wanted to make something special for Madhukar so decided to stop at the fish market. It took me longer than I expected to get home. I was burning with guilt thinking of my little girl shivering in the cold wintery air. Chitra was waiting for me on the front steps. Finally I reached home, parked the car in the garage and hurriedly ran upstairs hauling the grocery bags. As soon I opened the door, Chitra urged, "Aai, go upstairs to your bedroom."

"Can't you see the grocery bags in my hand, let me put the groceries away first?" I was a little edgy.

She pulled my sleeve, "No, no let's go upstairs."

I tried to remain calm as I followed her upstairs. She dragged me to our bedroom window and pointed down smilingly. On a carpet of white snow, the sticks and the twigs were arranged into "Happy Anniversary." Chitra got bored of waiting. Chitra's magic touch turned ordinary twigs sparked our yard into a beautiful warm greeting for us. I couldn't stop giving her hugs and kisses.

***

Swati kept her promise. She pushed away her weekends of leisure and started helping her mother, driving almost 70 miles round trip. Her mother didn't like clutter, so the first thing Swati would do as soon as she entered the house was to tidy up. She would insist that mother should go out and do something on her own, which of course her mother refused stubbornly. Swati inherited the love of poetry from her parents and would read poems that she came across to her mother. Then it was time to laugh at Swati's silly jokes; she took after her dad with her humor. She would always bring a book or an article for her mother to read. Quietly she would hide a little cherub or other small gift where mother would be least expecting it. So not only she took charge of her Dad but also nurtured her mother's spirit. One day she arrived for her usual Saturday morning mission.

When they had moved to this new house seven years ago, Jyoti had shoved all the stuff into the upstairs room, to take care of it later but that later never arrived. The office was packed with his books, published papers, tax documents, and Jyoti's writings, diaries, all the old magazines in which Jyoti was published, paints, paintings, and scraps of material from her sewing hobby. The pile of old LP records was stacked mutely in the middle of it all. In the corner was a bookshelf with rare collections of English/Marathi, Yoga, and philosophy books. They decided to tidy that room.

Jyoti was swamped to see how much she had collected. "If only Daddy and I didn't have any of these hobbies' life would have been lot simpler and this room wouldn't be so cluttered," she confessed.

"But Aai, your life would have been so boring," Swati promptly convinced her.

Jyoti was buried in the past while sorting through her old sketches… *'I remember that particular Sunday- Lokmanya Tilak's Jayanti. She started telling Swati. 'On the front page of the newspaper was his photo. I started to copy his picture on our blackboard. I felt Dada's pat on my shoulder, "Waa, waa, Jyo, what an exact image you drew! Don't wipe it, let's keep it in honor of our freedom fighter's birthday celebration." Dada's face was glowing with admiration for my drawing.*

After some time Visu Mama Narawane came. He was not truly related, but you know how it is. Like Madhukar used to say, at Deodhar's house they have Elmer's glue, and whoever comes to their home automatically become uncles or aunts. My Aai's brothers had all stayed at Dadar with us at one time. So their friends used to call your Aaji- tai-an elder sister and I would call them mama, maternal uncle. Visu Mama always pampered me, bringing me candies. When he saw my sketch, he picked me up and carried me triumphantly on his shoulder, running around the rooms, "Jyotiba, Jyotiba!"

Honestly, I had never liked being called a boy's name as I was definitely not a boy. "Jyotiba, one day we will have your painting exhibition in the famous Jahangir Art Gallery in the Fort area of Bombay!"

I was only seven years old. I had no idea what an art gallery was. I used to copy every picture that caught my eye. Drawing became my hobby. I didn't have colored crayons or pencils, yet I kept drawing. Sometimes Dada would frown at my constant scribblings.

Over summer vacation we were in Belgaum visiting Baba and Akka. We were playing Lagori with the neighboring children in the backyard. Suddenly the shrill siren of the train rang out. We stood frozen in the middle of the game, not knowing what had happened. The train station was nearby, and everybody started running towards it. The game was forgotten, and we children followed the crowd. There was a shattered body lying down on the tracks. Ushatai held my hand so tightly that it hurt. I could see she was frightened. She said, "Jyoti don't go there. He is dead." "Dead? What do you mean?"
My seven-year brain had no idea what death really was. I was not afraid. I jerked my hand from her grasp and started running to where the crowed was headed. When I approached at the dead body, I was stunned. His head was cracked and something that looked like a pink cauliflower was hanging out of it. I bent down to see it closely. I was fascinated by that sight, the first time in my life that I observed the inside of the human body. At that very moment, all that curiosity made me want to see even more of our bodies. "I am going to be a doctor when I grow up," I declared to Dada pompously when we returned to Dadar. Dada was thrilled. He started telling everybody with pride, "My daughter is going to be a doctor!" I was flattered by his praise, which was unknowingly brainwashing me.

Later I was fascinated by the pictures by my favorite artist, Dinanath Dalal. I started copying them along with other artists' work for practice. Once I was doodling something on my notebook, not really listening to Mrs. Nerurkarbai, our 8th grade teacher. She caught me red-handed and dashed over to me with fury, "Jyotsna why aren't you paying attention?" and snatched my notebook. I was afraid that I would be sent to the principal's office. She forgot to punish me and instead the words popped from her mouth, "Oh, how nice! Your sketch is really a masterpiece." Laughter erupted in the classroom.

In the same year I took two drawing exams just for fun. I used to enjoy drawing Rangolis and decorating our hands with mehndi. Childhood scurried away too quickly, and the final year approached. I buried myself in my studies. I would be taking all the science courses for college preparation. Summer vacation had just started. It was in the afternoon and my Aai and other ladies in our building were playing a game of bridge. Gajanan, Shanta Maushi's son, came for a visit. Aai told him to wait for few minutes, she would make some tea for him once she finished her game. He nodded and took a notebook from his Shabnam bag and quietly started sketching Aai.

I was fascinated by the speed of his fast-moving hand, his pen in full force. With only a few lines he captured Aai's spirit. I was speechless. Until then I had never seen anybody doing a sketch of a live person. Those lines entangled me into a fascinating new world. I didn't even realize that in that enchanting moment all the dreams of becoming a medical doctor evaporated. It was a turning point in my life. A magical door opened. I decided to follow in Gajanan's footsteps and join art school. The final exams results came, and I got distinction in my high school graduation. Dada told everybody as he was passing around pedhas (a typical sweet one distributes after getting good news), "Now Jyoti is going to fulfill my dream. She is going to become a doctor!"

I could not bear to see his disappointment when I told him about my change of heart. Only with Aai and Aba's full support was I able to gather my courage even though Dada could not give me his blessings.

Until I attended the J.J. School of Art my blindness had stopped me from appreciating the abundant beauty present in everyday life. Sometimes, even in the emptiness of a void I would see a beautiful sculpture. This was truly a spiritual intimate experience for me. I was intoxicated by the sheer joy of art. In spite of achieving scholarships throughout all 4 years, Dada would still beg me, "Jyo, there is still time, you would easily get admission to medical school."

Dada came to our house in Framingham for the very first time when you girls were young. As soon as he entered the house he exclaimed, "No doubt this house belongs to an artist!"

Dada's praise dwarfed all the prizes from my exhibitions. Listening to his words was my highest honor. Yet the splinter kept digging deep inside me that I never fulfilled Dada's wish for me to become a doctor. If I had listened to his advice, I would have been financially independent, earning my own living. I sold lots of paintings, but I knew that I was not able to support myself on my art alone without Madhukar's full and enthusiastic backing and financial support.

I used to wonder in my college days where all these ideas were coming to me for my paintings. Sometimes my ego would balloon up and I would assume that the inspiration came only from myself. Then I heard from Dada that his grandfather had been an artist who used to do murals on the temple's walls. All the creativity that I was caressing tightly as my own was actually inherited from my ancestors. After listening to Vimalaji Thakar's lectures, I found out that it comes not just from ancestors but from the land you live on, the culture you have known, the nature around you. Swat, did you know Dada used to write poetry? Every time I visited Aaji in Pune; she would surprise me reciting his poems. All this I found out much later in my adulthood.

My Aai knew about the art of living and was very creative in everyday life. She always tried something different while cooking. She was appreciative of the nature around her. She would stand in her gallery and watch the birds tenderly. She always had some flowers on her table. One time when I arrived in Pune, I noticed that she drew a rangoli on the threshold to welcome me. She fondly remembered that once on her birthday I had drawn a traditional rangoli around her dinner plate. I asked her why she never did any of these artsy things in Dadar? Her simple answer, "I never had my own house or the time." Her words were spoken without bitterness.

"Aai, all that's true but then you would have been a miserable doctor," Swati's tight embrace, brought Jyoti back in the room. They both started to tidy up the room. But the more they sorted Madhukar's books and notes, the more they were tempted to keep it all. Swati was not surprised at his collection of intellectual books, but she became overwhelmed once again being reminded of her father's academic achievements and his vast knowledge. She was used to the shining rays of his intellect since her childhood. It was taken for granted all this time. But now all that was wiped away by his Alzheimer's.

"Did you know, anybody who had difficulty in their studies or work would always come to him. They knew he would have the right answer and would never make anybody feel inferior or humiliated, including me. I used to call him my talking encyclopedia. Of course, this was before Google kī jai!" Jyoti's voice was heavy with gratitude. The thought of how much had changed, all his research papers and lectures no longer current, devastated Swati. Reluctantly she carried all his books to her car to donate to a local library or book drop.

In her last few visits, Swati noticed that her Daddy was not talking at all and mentioned this to her Aai. "What can I say, Swati, he stopped talking almost a month ago. I didn't want you girls to feel sad, so I stayed mute. I am blessed with two wonderful caring daughters. I don't know what I would have done without you two angels. Her eyes were teary with gratitude. She could not bear the thought that her daughters would no longer have their loving father's shelter. The clock didn't know how long the mother and daughter locked themselves in a comforting hug. The room filled with a silence that echoed with all the harsh reality of their life. Jyoti noticed that evening Swati was unusually quiet. After taking her father to bed, they both watched an artsy movie which Swati had brought specially for her mother. Still, sadness lingered in their mind.

The next morning, Jyoti woke up and got breakfast ready. Madhukar was always ravenous in the morning. She peeked into Swati's room, but her bed was empty. Assuming Swati must have gone for a morning walk, she hurried to his room. She couldn't miss the dried tears on Swati's cheeks, sleeping next to her father as if she were his little girl again. She was tempted to bask in the sunshine of the happy days, when the girls would jump in their bed to cuddle up on a Sunday morning with giggles and make a sandwich between them.

***

September 9, 2011

"Aai, I am going to come with you to the lawyer's office", Chitra announced as soon as she noticed the date on my calendar. I was amazed by her observation. I had not even mentioned it to her. I couldn't help but admire her thoughtfulness. When did this little girl grew up so fast, to be such a successful career woman? Not just a CPA but Director of Finance of her company in such a short time. She is efficient and knowledgeable in practical matters in everyday life. With her ever-demanding job I didn't want to bother her with one additional responsibility. I knew she had a deadline coming up soon. She had to drive an hour to work and came home late in the evening. Never complained. I knew there was no point trying to change her mind about accompanying me. I opened the car door to sit next to her. Shopping bags were piled up on the seat. "What did you buy?" I asked out of curiosity.

"Oh, nothing much. When I go to work in the morning, I see a lot of homeless people begging at the traffic light. My heated seat comforts me in the car but made me wonder how those people suffer in the cold weather. So I bought these for them. Instead of giving them money, I hand them hats and mittens and granola bars."

She told me this as a matter of fact. "Chit, I am so proud of your acts of kindness." She made my day.

Until then Madhukar used to take care of all our taxes, investments, and legal issues. Now Chitra had taken over, including these back-and-forth trips to the lawyer's office for the last few weeks. Everything was pretty much under control with our trust. Today we just needed to finalize a few last things, so we brought Madhukar along to sign some papers, which was a difficult task for him. Our lawyer was aware of his impairments, but she was extremely impressed by his foresight of taking out long-term care insurance for both of us. Because of him I would not have to worry in my old age.

***

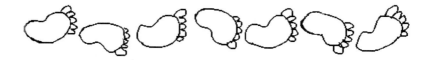

Every child is an artist. The problem is how to remain an artist once we grow up. - Pablo Picasso

February 4, 2012

I was in Boston's Museum of Fine Arts after a long time. I was in seventh heaven in that ambiance. I saw an old painting of Degas and took a step back to gaze at it from a distance. I accidentally bumped into somebody behind me. "Oh, I am so sorry!" I apologized to a young man behind me.

He smiled and casually said to me, "Have a nice day." "You too," I smiled back at him and reciprocated with the same, didn't know if he heard me since he had moved on to another painting. Such simple ordinary words! But his greetings touched me deeply and carved on my heart. My mind became a little tender yet pensive by his kind words and I was taken back by my strong reaction.

Last week when Paul at the pool asked me, "How are you, Jyoti? I have not seen you for a long time." His caring question filled me the same pleasant feeling. But the very next minute I became teary. Those gentle words turned into a sharp arrow wounding my heart. I was so focused on Madhukar, that I had forgotten that somebody could care about my own wellbeing…

It had been more than a year since Madhukar started firing his fury at me. His shouting had ruptured my mind so deeply that I was worried the walls of our house would get cracked by his hammering shouts. Over the months his rage progressed even more. Madhukar and I were each other's mirror until then. We could see each other's minds clearly, read each other's thoughts instantly. We were each other's best friends. But now I have been exiled from his caring dialogs. My mind was often bewildered. Who was this stranger I was living with? Definitely not my Raja. Deprived of his tender love, I became orphaned. The reality hit me hard and I became desperately hungry for kindness. I started sucking on those mundane greetings – 'Have a nice day', 'How are you?' like candy from proper strangers. My days didn't include friendly simple chats with anybody. My world was made only of doctors, pharmacists, insurance companies, caregivers, and lawyers. All my friends were on a different path in the distance. I no longer had the urge or strength to pick up the phone and have a heart-to-heart chat with people who were once my friends.

Madhukar was already at the third stage out of five when he was diagnosed with Alzheimer's. It had affected not just his cognitive abilities but his speech also. It slowly robbed him of his evergreen personality. *I cannot even imagine the way this imposed muteness must be screaming in his mind. Is he aware of all this in his heart? How restless he must be with agony of the unknown.* A brush fire leaping from one question to another. turning into anguished blaze. Then I heard on the news that the famous singer Glen Campbell also became a victim of this disease. His concerts would cease now. Listening to his last song, I pictured Madhukar up there on the stage singing for me.

The sounds in my mind never emerge into words anymore.

I will never wipe away the dust of your worries. Do you know who I am? I don't know you but my love for you will remain forever. Forever.

Selfish I am indeed. I don't even think of your being. Your face, our daughter's giggles, your tears, your wounded heart. I do not see them anymore. Selfish I am indeed. You are vanished from my mind forever...

The young man that I bumped into was my angel for the day. His gentle words doused the fire from my mind, making me relaxed. I carried that peace with me for a long time passing through the hallways of the museum when suddenly another angel appeared on the wall in front of me. Two paintings by Picasso. One was a realistically depicted image of a clown, and the other was a more abstract, cubist portrait of a woman. Joy flowered all over me. I untangled the twisted shattered pieces of her face and was able to see the real beauty. I first saw prints of this painting in a book in the library at art school. Instantly Picasso became my mentor. His paintings and sculptures have penetrated deep down into my own art.

Picasso must have known of my devotion because he would always lure us, wherever we were. It was 1988 and we were roaming in Lucerne, Switzerland. Suddenly it started raining like cats and dogs, catching us unguarded. We were looking for a shelter and saw an art museum. It pulled us like a magnet and without a word we started walking towards its entrance. There was Picasso again, his rare paintings on display. We saw a documentary on his life; he had so many hobbies and pets (goats, pigeons, dogs). I was grateful to the showers for this hidden treasure.

Later when we were in Vienna, the same thing happened. There was a huge exhibition on Picasso. His peaceful dove was created for the United Nations. Until then I was not aware of his strong political views.

We were on a flight to Madrid. Looking at a tour guide that I was reading, a fellow passenger started talking to me about what to see there. I expressed my disappointment that since we were not going to Barcelona, I wouldn't get to see Picasso's famous Guernica. He informed me that Guernica had actually been transferred to Madrid's art museum. Madhukar said of course we will have to see it. When we landed, we threw our luggage in the hotel room, ignored our jet lag, and rushed to the bus to the museum. We hurried to Picasso's hall. Guernica, that huge painting, stood strong. It occupied the entire wall from one end to the other. I just stood there mesmerized by it. I was speechless with all it was saying to me. The war! No matter how small or big, the atrocities of war are felt by generations after generations. Picasso had expressed without colors only in black and white, still so heart wrenchingly. You can't escape the brutality without feeling sad, and I was not an exception to that.

I do not support any kind of war between people or nations. I know even a glorious victory comes with a price to pay; this has been known since the Mahabharata war.

"Would you pick up a weapon to defend America if the time came?"

I flatly denied the question and check marked it in the big "NO" column and finished the questionnaire for citizenship. I prepared myself for the outcome. Obviously, they would deny me citizenship if I refused to fight.

I was still in awe over Guernica. Forty-one years back when I studied Picasso in college, I never dreamed that one day I would see this painting in person. This encounter was nothing but a Sakshatkar. Unknowingly my hands joined in humble namaskar. The tears started streaming into a garland of gratitude, I just bent down and kept bowing to Picasso and his Guernica over and over again like I was in the temple.

***

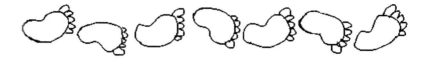

Live as the will of God but remember to have contentment -
Saint Tukaram

January 16, 2013

Every time I went to the caregiver's workshop, the director kept telling me, "Don't forget to keep open communication with your daughters and to ask them for help. Remember, he is their father." Having communication with them was no difficulty but to ask for help even from my own daughters was indeed hard for me. As it is, I knew that they were extremely sad to face their father's condition. So I did not want them to have this illness's shadow overpowering their life more. Why bother them with extra burden? So I tried to take care of Madhukar as much as I could. Besides, they were always helping me by going out of their way to cheer me up. Swati, Chit, Mark, and Jeevan had always been there for me.

Like today, both of them had already decided they were going to have a date with their daddy, DDD (Daddy Daughters Day) and that I was going to spend some time with Jeevan at the Museum of Fine Arts in Boston.

Green lights at the signal gave a nod to this pilgrimage. I was on my way to my muse. I hurriedly parked the car in an empty spot right in front of the museum and fed some coins to the machine. Jeevan and I started galloping toward the main entrance. Many days-months-years had passed since I was here last time! The bitter cold wind of January stung through to my bones. I assured myself that all the art inside would make me warm. This love affair between art museum and I was ancient. It started in art school and later Madhukar and I cultivated this passion ever since we got married.

When we moved to Boston, I was delighted to find the MFA. I still remember that first day. Like a little girl I skipped down the steps of the library as soon as I got the museum pass. The visit would be short since I had to come back before the girls returned from school that afternoon.

"Long time no seen. Where have you been?" The Native American chief sitting astride his horse became momentarily alive and winked at me. Jeevan startled me as he was pulling my sleeves, "Aaji, the chief is looking at you!"

"Aaji, look at all those birds."

"Canadian geese, my favorite!" I felt nostalgic. The flapping of their wings flew my mind back many years. I started telling Jeevan...Our very first house in 1969 was on a little pond in Framingham. My first fall in New England. One day I heard a loud honking, so I ran outside to see a huge flock of birds landing on the water. A carpenter was working on our roof, and he shouted, "I am going to shoot this fat Canadian goose for Thanksgiving dinner." How could he even think of killing them? I was horrified. I yelled back at him, "Not from my yard!"

I fell in love with those 'exotic' birds. I wished I could also migrate like them back to sunny Mumbai. Graceful white necks, yellow beaks, black and white lines on their gray wings were so mesmerizingly elegant! I didn't even know when I captured the goose on my canvas that same afternoon. Jeevan, do you remember that painting? Swati Maushi has it.

Jeevan nodded and started walking with me, taking interest in our tour. I was proud of Jeevan and grateful that he was really interested in art. We spent hours lingering at each painting at the museum. My body, my mind felt alive again in this inspiring environment. This was a rare opportunity for Grandson and his Aaji, hand in hand, to appreciate the paintings while the daughters were taking care of their Daddy, who was now beyond art and other joys of this world.

"Jeevan, Ajoba and I used to come here very often; he was very much interested in art," I murmured. I wanted him to remember

Ajoba's good old days. Jeevan was the apple of his eye. How he used to play with him, take him for walks in the stroller, feed him, read books to him at bedtime. But Jeevan does not remember any of that pampering that ended when he was only four years of age.

Now Jeevan pushes Ajoba's wheelchair, teaches him how to hold the spoon at dinner table. All he sees now is silent Ajoba, not able to utter a single word, angrily slapping him once in a while for no reason; this from a father who never once spanked his own daughters. It was heartbreaking for me to think that Jeevan would not know Ajoba's vibrant enthusiasm for life. My mind lingered on Madhukar's lively personality.

Colors from the painting in front of me faded away. The gallery walls closed upon me. Turmoil flooded over me. "How can I go on 24x7 caring for Madhukar? Putting the suppository in, feeding, bathing him, and dressing him. The list went on. His dignity was robbed while his illness sucked away my muses too. Lately he was falling a lot, which I could not handle physically. My own inability defeated me completely. I realized that I too had stopped living. I couldn't remember the last time I took a paint brush in hand to lose myself on the canvas. My body and mind were dry as a bone, a riverbed in scorching summer.

But that day in the museum I felt alive again. The entire ambiance nourished my soul like a parched vine thrives in the rain. Creativity flowed in my veins making me alive again. For a moment I was able to separate myself from my beloved. I was a stranger to this long-lost freedom. All the inspiration rushed in my blood and I flourished again.

We returned to Swatu's apartment around 3 p.m. in the afternoon. All of a sudden, I felt very fatigued, and my back was hurting. All the stress I had endured since Madhukar was diagnosed with Alzheimer's stormed in my mind. I had no idea how tired and utterly exhausted I was. For a year now, his doctor was constantly telling me to find a nursing home, advice I was deaf to. My mind would taunt "You already lost him when he became a victim of Alzheimer's."

A year ago I tried to take Madhukar to a nearby day care center.

When the secretary at the daycare started her list of questions to evaluate him, Madhukar got very frustrated and annoyed.

"Let's leave this place, I don't like it here," his voice hissed full of venom.

He was rushing to the door already. I was planning to take him back again. So the next day instead of going to the pool, I drove my car on the same road toward the day care center.

"Where are we heading? I know where you are taking me. I am not going back there again," he roared like a wild beast. I was shocked to see his instant reaction. How did he even register that I changed the route?

I was terrified; what if he became violent and hit me while I was driving? The scary tales that I had heard repeatedly in the support group seemed about to happen to me. I obediently turned the car toward Holiday Inn's pool in silence. But today I realized that I was hanging onto a hope so fragile that it finally broke with all the weight I had been carrying around. Maybe some fresh air would help. I left Swati apartment in hurry. A new hidden road opened in my mind on that walk. Even though that path was more difficult and thornier than the one I was currently on. I realized I couldn't do this anymore. I confessed and accepted the reality. No smooth ride was left.

***

January 17, 2013

"Raja, we are going to follow Dr. Khera's advice. She said we need to give some creative challenges to stimulate your brain. In the center they have many ways to keep you occupied. So we are going to try it tomorrow, okay?"

After she had told him this yesterday evening, he just sat there, eyes vacant and drawn toward the ceiling. She consoled herself that his lack of reaction was because he had always respected Dr. Khera's treatment in the past. Still his passiveness stabbed at her.

Break of dawn. She knew what lay ahead today. She put a lid on her thoughts and started getting him ready. Without a word, she turned her car towards the Mansfield Day Care Center. She was preparing herself with a shield of courage to face his resistance and hostility, but that morning he did not recognize the route. He stayed quiet, didn't utter even a word. His silence defeated her.

She parked the car at the center. Helped him to get out and held his hand firmly, guiding him to the front entrance. He started walking slowly along with her quiet as a snail. Yesterday she had called the center to inform them that she would be bringing him this morning, and the nurse was ready to welcome him. She took him to the TV room. He joined the group without protest. Did he really like her idea, or could he not figure out the situation?

"Raja, I will be back soon to pick you up. Enjoy all the activities until then," she promised him. Before her mind could change, she controlled her tears and hurriedly entrusted him to their friendly care. She escaped through the door like a wounded prey from the hunter. Tons of burden disappeared from her shoulders. She remembered giving the same assurance to Swati on her very first day of nursery school so many years ago. She came home with hundreds of ideas about how to spend her day, but she ended up just sipping hot ginger tea and reading Time magazine leisurely and without interruption.

Although she turned her car towards the pool, the wheels took her home instead with a heavy heart. Not only was she just a mother for eternity, but a wife for everlasting time. She felt the house was barren. Usually her abode would blanket her in a serene comfort, but today it only gave her the feeling of being orphaned. She was preoccupied in keeping an eye on Madhukar. She was constantly fastened to him like his shadow. Today that shadow felt desolate. She had all the time in the world but couldn't find the way to do her mind's desire. She was so lost without him. She dialed the phone… "Hello."

"Dr. Jangi here." When Dr. Khera could not care for Madhukar's illness, Jyoti found respite in Rohit Jangi's help. He was a geriatric expert and happily - but sadly - took over Madhukar's care. Rohit had great admiration for Madhukar. When he first came to see Madhukar after his illness began, Rohit was heartbroken to see his condition.

"Rohit, I enrolled Madhukar in the adult day care center today." She still could not believe her own words.

"That's great! How did you manage it? I am really proud of you, Jyoti."

"There is nothing to be proud of. This is nothing but a weakness, a sheer defeat, a failure, a desperation," she confessed through her sobbing.

***

She didn't want Madhukar to get rebellious, so she went to pick up him up after only two hours. The nurse told him that he was indeed devastated. He became very teary instantly as soon as she left and started asking every person like a lost child,

"Where is my wife? Have you seen my wife? Where did she go?"
Then he just sat near the door. As soon as he saw her enter, he ran to her like a little boy. He hugged her again and again, clinging to her. His tearful revelation, "Jyoti, I really missed you. I kept thinking of you. Where were you?"

She was stunned…These cascades of words, where were they coming from? Even though they were full of sadness, her thirsty spirit was happy to be drenched under that shower. Her guilt gnawing at her as she was going to continue this. Next day she kept him there from 10:00 am to 2:30 pm.

***

February 4, 2013

She was glad to realize that Michelle from the support group was right. Madhukar was getting used to day care. He still referred to it as a prison, though, and immediately she would try to assure him, "You mean school. One doesn't come home every day from prison, Raja."

Weeks went by. He was indeed getting used to the routine. When he woke every morning, the first thing he would ask her, "Are we going there?" and then without any grumbling he would get ready with her help.

Sometimes when she was picking him up, he was not willing to come home, and she wondered if he was beginning to forget his home.

"So what did you do today at the center?" she asked him on the way home.

"Don't interrogate me like a court," he snapped at her suddenly.

That same afternoon she picked up Jeevan from school on the way. At the dinner table she asked her usual, "What did you do at school today, Jeevan? What was your high today?"

Jeevan enthusiastically popped out the answer, "Aaji, you know! Coming here is always my high! School was lot of fun. I enjoyed my art class today."

Madhukar immediately said, "I took part in all the things today."

She was stunned by his instant response; just a while ago he had resisted telling her that in the car. She could tell he was getting used to and liking the adult day care center. She silently prayed to the Goddess to let this continue and to please give her the strength to take care of him.

***

March 15, 2013

At the breakfast table she would read aloud from her 'Daily Thoughts' book. Today was no exception. In the commentary after the day's quote the author asked, "Whom would you like to spend your life with?"

Madhukar instantly replied, "With Jyoti." These moments were rare like a dance of fireflies in the foggy night. No way of telling what his behavior was going to be day by day. Two months had gone by now. She still felt as if she were stumbling in the dark always. She walked into the daycare to see what he was doing. He was sitting on the chair facing against the door, rubbing his hands harshly. This obsessive rubbing hands was getting out of control, as was his confusion growing like wild grass. Lately she was extremely worried that he was forgetting her also. He kept turning his head back and forth toward the door. She could easily sense that he was restless. She went as quietly as a cat and stood behind his chair. She covered his eyes and whisper in his ears, "Can you guess who this is?"

Without a moment's delay, the words slid out of his mouth, "Jyoti! Jyoti, my wife for the last 46 years!"

Her mind glided on a jubilant rainbow of delight, as if she had found the same colorful kaleidoscope that Dada had once bought for her at the fair. Just as the glass pieces disappear in its lenses and one only sees a labyrinth of beautifully colorful designs. Her heart was shattered from his unbearable suffering. But all those thousand pieces of her anguish disappeared, and his words kept appearing over and over in the kaleidoscope of her mind. But all that joy lasted only for a second before it was extinguished by his vacant eyes as he turned away from her in muteness. He walked into the other room, indifferently turning his back to her as if she were a proper stranger. After she put the seatbelt on him, she placed a bunch of long-stemmed yellow roses on his lap. He used to bring her flowers all the time. He picked up the bunch and kept smelling the roses until they reached home.

Nowadays, he was behaving like an innocent child. He would mimic her often. She used to tease him often in the past, "Do you know why god made me a preschool teacher? So I can train my dear husband."

Before, when they went for walks, she had a hard time keeping up with his pace, making her run seven steps behind him. But all that had changed. His walk became too slow and that lingering walk would hurt her back. So today she asked Ellie to take him for a walk instead and decided to go for a brisk solo walk. Ellie held his hand and guided him out of the door. He didn't like holding her hand; He unfolded her grip, looked at her intensely, and without a word held her hand again and started dragging his feet. Sometimes he would favor Ellie as if she were his daughter Chitra. Lately Jyoti noticed that he was having a hard time with English and was speaking only in Marathi. He would grumble at Ellie, "Why don't you speak in Marathi to me?"

As she was on her second walk around the neighborhood, she saw them in the distance. As he came near to her, he almost waved his hand, a little wrinkle of smile sprouted on his face. She went closer and touched his hand. The softness of his palm gave her a solid reassurance and the words start trotting as they went again in opposite directions.

I am madly in love with you.
Your hand swaying towards me in the air,
I fall in love with you all over again.
At the next corner,
again you hold your hand up,
giving me a sure sign of old friendship,
and bringing my hopes high.
But as I come closer to you, you walk away in your own world.
Your eyes never show me any trace that we only just met few minutes before.
Our paths cross again.
You stand still momentarily and try to extend your hand.
Your hand brushes my hand expecting it to be held.
Puckering your lips, you allow me to kiss you right there on the corner.
I hold on to this precious moment close to my heart.

When I come to the next corner,
your eyes shine for a split second. Your smile is vague.
Still I fall for you all over again.
I am madly in love again. I am madly in love again with you.

A faint signal in your eyes gives me a receipt of our past closeness. You pull me back through the corridors of years after years. They say, in this illness, the past memory is intact. So I tease you, poking an old memory of our first meeting, and ask you the same question you had asked me that day, "Have we met before?"

The same words that you uttered to me in the restaurant Resham Bhavan rebounded in my mind. Only this time we were in Chicago. Your work meeting was finished earlier than expected. I was returning to the hotel from the Art Institute and you bumped into me at the corner. Our eyes caressed each other lovingly. A rare confession slipped through your locked lips, "I am quite sure that we have met before in the past. But today, seeing you again, I fell in love with you all over again."
Forty-six years have whisked by since then. But that old memory… the fragrance of Bakul flowers is still very fresh in my mind. At the dinner table, I light a candle. The stereo is playing the evening rag Marawa. The microwave hums and then the shrilling rings of the phone. I get annoyed by some telemarketer trying to sell me something, yell at them, "Leave me alone!"

I start instructing Elly about your night care. Finally I am done feeding you. So too ends the Marawa. Elly takes charge of you. I am about to sit down for my dinner with a sigh of relief, "How peaceful it is!" The words slip out of my lips.

"Because you stopped talking," you erupt with those words.

Laughter burst out of my throat from your spontaneous humor; your comment gave me the satisfaction of a feast before I even begin eating. A dance of a firefly in a foggy night continues.

"Good night Irene, Good night Irene, I'll see you in my dreams" I am humming the lullaby.

The afternoon sun shone high in the sky stamping out the shadows beneath my feet. I finished lunch and then tried to juggle a few more chores around the house. I had a couple of hours before getting Madhukar from the center. I was tempted to do Shavasan, but in the middle of my relaxation, the phone startled me. I saw the caller ID of his center. Nurse Eileen was on the phone, "Jyoti, you better come right away. You need to take Dr. J to his doctor. He has a temperature of 106."

'Oh, my god!' I left the house with a jolt. How did this happen? Such a high temperature! I might have to take him to the emergency room. Is this another symptom of Alzheimer's? I didn't remember reading that in the book. If the fever goes high, he could go into shock. Why didn't they call an ambulance right away? The questions swarmed. I tried to focus on my breathing while I was driving, telling myself that I might not even see him again. Prepare yourself; nobody knows what destiny has in store. When Baba died, his best friend who was an expert palmist was shocked to hear about his untimely death. He never saw it coming. 'Bhagawati, if this is his last moment, please don't make him suffer more. Please help him and let his further journey be peaceful and please protect him', I began to pray continuously. 'Raja, you know I always loved you to death. Our love story would go forever. Don't worry, I will follow you immediately.' The four miles stretched like four hundred miles. I raced to the center. To my surprise, Madhukar was sitting calmly and watching TV. I was relieved but extremely baffled. I ran to Eileen, "How did his temperature rocket so high?" She looked at me in doubt, "100.6 is not so high! But I still think he should be seen by the doctor, just in case."

I realized that I had heard it wrong. My mind began to calm down, teaching me a firm lesson. *Idam na mam. Idam na mam.* This is not mine. Let it go. Let it go.

***

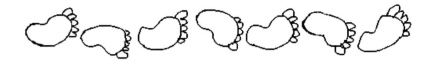

Strength doesn't come from physical capacity. It comes from an indomitable will. – Mahatma Gandhi

December 22, 2012

The Nepali vendor was sitting on the footpath trying to sell his antique silver oxide jewelry. She was trying to get a good bargain on a ring. She was drawn by its big, round, turquoise stone. Finally she gave in and emptied all the loose coins from her purse into his hands. She admired the ring on her finger and started walking towards Jahangir Art gallery. That whole day the turquoise kept caressing not just her finger but her mind too. But as soon as she got home that evening, Dada scolded, "Take that ring off your finger. Where did you get it? Don't you know that is the stone of malicious Saturn?"

His roar put a damper on her. Without a word of protest, the ring slid from her finger. Silently but cunningly she put it in her purse without Dada noticing. The next day as she approached the college, she slipped the ring back again onto her finger. On the way home she took it off. This became her clever routine. Many years passed by. One day she was mesmerized again by the same turquoise color when Madhukar returned from Arizona with some native jewelry. A really valuable turquoise ring for her and some earrings for the girls. The turquoise captivated her with the joy of a peacock's dance. Later when they were in Sedona, she was convinced that her fascination came from one of her past lives, and that she must have been Native American. On another trip to a Tekadi resort in South India, Madhukar surprised her with a string of exclusive turquoise beads. From then on, she wore all the turquoise jewelry with fondness and without inhibition.

She blinks her eyes; just a moment ago she was swinging on the blue-green waves. She had seen that unusual color of the sea for the first time in 1967 in Beirut. That was their first stop from Bharat to America and was part of their European honeymoon. She had lost herself watching the dance of the waves from the window of their hotel room. The artist in her could not decide if that color was aquamarine or turquoise.

Now she pondered whether that gem of Saturn had brought this catastrophe on her. She was never a believer of superstitions. After her marriage to Madhukar, she found out that the Joshi family they didn't worship Lord Ganesh because his wrath was very fierce towards them. She was dismayed to learn that. How could Ganesh or any deity be angry at his/her devotees? She was used to worshipping him, the savior from all difficulties and problems. Ever since she could remember there were huge weeklong celebrations of Ganesh's birthday in Narayan Niwas. Their small apartment would be full of visitors for darshan of Ganesh, and the ambience of bhakti was abundant. Chanting of bhajans and kirtans was so joyful. She would be sad when it was time for visarjan of the clay idol. She was baffled by how this could all change overnight just because she became a Joshi. Later when they had their own apartment in Decatur, she still could not go against her mother-in-law's warning. She only celebrated Ganesh's birthday by offering sweet coconut filled modaks, which her girls loved. She kept collecting little statues of Ganesh, but only as a decoration and never for worshipping. But today, all her firm belief in Ganesh's blessing began to tremor. Or was it, Saturn who has his Vakrdrushti, his evil eye, on Madhukar? She was saddened to think that because of her not following the rules, Madhukar was being punished with this cruel disease. All the doubts turned into sharp arrows that wounded her heart deeply. She locked that beautiful shade of greenish blue in the deepest chamber of her heart and threw away her warm quilt. She started her day with a stark mind.

First, she put the kettle on for tea. Then takes Madhukar to the bathroom. Today it seems like the kettle is impatient and starts whistling shrieking all over the house that the water is boiling. She can't leave him alone in the bathroom anymore. He would lose his balance. Her one foot starts going towards the kitchen and the other stumbles with him. Her usual juggling while walking on a tight rope. She measures his sugar and reading the number on the meter, her heart skips a beat. Oh my god, 20? How can it be? Something is wrong. She doesn't want to take any chances. So she runs to the kitchen and brings him a tablespoon of sugar to eat. She can't allow him to get hypoglycemic. After a while he is sitting on the chair again, and she starts getting his breakfast ready. He seems ok, but she decides to measure his sugar again.

The thought of piercing a needle into his finger stabs her more than the actual drop of blood; he himself is not bothered by this. 160. The number is a little higher than usual, but it is better than having hypo. She is finally sitting down to sip her hot ginger chai. Her sigh of relief is startled by the ringing phone. Who is calling this early in the morning? Her eyebrows frown, but then the smile curls up when she sees the caller ID of Swati. "Aai, I have taken a day off today. Let's go out for lunch. I wanted to tell you before you get ready for swimming. How is Daddy? Let me say hi to him. You come here to JP. I know you like to roam around here looking at the shops."

She treasures these moments like precious pearls, her darling daughter surprises to cheer her up. She hurriedly gets him ready with a sudden surge of energy and they're on their way to Jamaica Plain. It took 40 minutes to reach the parking lot. Her nostrils fill up with the aroma of Indian cooking. It has been so long since she was here last time. She had totally forgotten that Bukhara, the famous restaurant of Kashmiri cuisine, is just across the street. The menu on the chalkboard outside is mouthwatering. But she avoids the temptation and holds Madhukar's hand tightly to cross the street. She sees Swati running toward them. Swati loops both of them in a tight hug and unlocks Aai's grip of her father's hand and takes charge of him. While walking along the sidewalk Jyoti spots the sign for Café Beirut. "Oh, I remember reading a great review about this in The Boston Globe. Swati, let's try it."

She notices a charming girl at the counter. Her olive skin, sharp nose, and deep brown eyes decorated with Kohl, definitely a middle eastern beauty. The girl greets her with an accent to stamp her nationality. Jyoti immediately asks, "Are you from Lebanon?" The girl nods shyly. "Oh, I fell in love with your Beirut when we were there 46 years ago! The turquois water of the Mediterranean Sea was so enchanting. I was strictly vegetarian then so could not do justice to your cuisine. Today will be another story. Tell me what's your specialty."

Moussaka, Baba ghanoush, lamb curry for Daddy... Swati and she order according to the girl's suggestions. Jyoti eats everything as if she were starving and before they are even finished, Swati orders the Baklava; she knows her mother's sweet tooth very well. They all are enjoying this heavenly feast. She imagines taking her time with each bite of baklava laden with honey syrup, but Madhukar suddenly becomes fidgety. She knows what that means. He needs to go to the toilet. His enlarged prostate puts pressure on him. But nowadays he can't manage it by himself. She always has to assist him in the bathroom. It takes him forever to urinate. She worries, 'He won't be able to cope in this unfamiliar place. He won't be able to go there alone. He will lose his composure and be extremely disturbed.' From now on she will have to go with him into public restrooms. She locks his hand in hers and guides him through the crowd, avoiding people's eyes. Luckily, it is a unisex bathroom. He gets very uptight seeing her standing right there next to him.

"Don't worry Raja, I will turn toward the wall, my back to you. So it will give you complete privacy." She had never before stayed so close to him like that at home. He is not able to express it, but this frustrates him, making him more confused. After much coaxing he finally finishes his business, while she is unknowingly holding her breath. He lets her clean him without any rebellion. She washes his and her hands silently. They come back to the table. He starts stuffing the remaining food into his mouth, forgetting he just had a whole meal. She has lost her appetite; the taste buds have turned into barbs. The salad starts wilting. The moussaka becomes tasteless. She tries her best to hide her nausea and tells Swati how delicious it was. Swati announces that they should put an order in for their New Year's Eve celebration. Her mind starts snarling, 'What is there to celebrate? This year has brought nothing but a terrible uphill turn to our life.'

Swati suggested they should walk inside Chestnut Hill Mall. Usually she avoids malls. Walking on those hard floors there hurts her back and she doesn't get pleasure out of window shopping amongst all the harried customers. But Chestnut Hill mall was much smaller, and the stores have class. "Aai, there is a nice art gallery just around the corner. Why don't you visit it? I will take Daddy for a walk and we can meet in an hour at Starbuck's."

One entire free hour? Her heart jumped temptingly of that break. As soon as she entered the gallery, her weary mind flourished. Her admiration for her daughter - she always knew how to boost her up - mixed with the art around her. Her lingering feet, appreciating all the sculptures and paintings, stilled at a collage on the wall. Her eyes narrowed on the seascape that the artist had created out of simple material. Bluish greenish peacock feathered color was concealed under the foam of white cotton. Far away above the turquoise waves there was a dark gray rough wool spread into a horizon. A hint of coming night. A lonely cloud of white cotton in the corner was still lingering, shadowing a dark mass on the waves. She could not figure out what the material was that the artist used for that shadow. Her depressed mind floated in that shadow. A collage appeared in front of her. Chitra had insisted that her Aai should do something for her headboard when they moved into a new house. She had painted Persian blue waves on a white malmal cotton with just a hint of turquoise. Then she added moon beams and sea foam on those waves using Chithra's silver painjan, a silver kargota (a girdle-like ornament tied around the waists of infants), her own silver zumkas that she had worn in her youth, refusing to give them up to Dada's approval. The last touch was silver sequins on the dark sky.

She had been very excited for her first grandchild's birth. When it was time to bring Jeevan home from the hospital, a very joyous Indian traditional entrance for the baby to his home, wearing his grandfather's homemade hooded baby blanket, she didn't have anything from his paternal Ajoba, but that didn't stop her. She decided to make a special quilt to wrap him in, using all the pieces from the maternal side. A cloth from her mother's 9-yard Induri sari, her Ashtputri sari (another tradition -the yellow Kanjiwaram silk wedding sari was given by her maternal uncle), Swati maushi's shawl, and Chit's wedding blouse. Whatever she could get her hands on. Their love was sewn into that blanket as if they were hugging him.

From then on, she kept collecting all the rags from whatever she sewed, feathers she found on her walks, gold and silver borders from her old saris…All that material she would use for her future collages. But now it is smothered in the old trunks which are kept in captivity in the attic. Just like all her motivation was stuck in her muddy mind. In the barren terrain of her mind, nothing grows anymore. She moaned, her mind drowned in tears, 'My creativity has been stolen along with Madhukar's memory. After all, he is my muse, my Sun and Moon. He always encouraged me to be productive in my creativity.' Suddenly that collage in front of her soared her back to a different cosmos. Her creativity sprouted again. She proclaimed to herself, 'I have always cradled this blessing of creativity so close to my bosom. I shall keep this inspiration alive.' Mantra begins to chant. 'Bloom in spite of all the storms lighting and thundering. Don't allow famine to conquer your hungers. You must remain loyal to your art!'

"This will be the perfect gift, fit for my Raja." She makes a resolution for the coming new year, to keep her promise to Dada that she would always use art in her everyday life. Her business cards start dancing in front of her eyes. Artful Living!!! The doubt in her mind bursts like a bubble. The artist in her awakens. Squeezing a tube, she covers the dark shadow in that collage with a vibrant turquoise. She steps out of the gallery with unusual strength and walks towards the coffee shop.

***

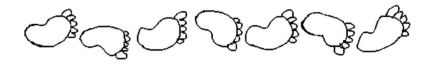

Kaya nahi teri, nahi teri. Mat kaho meri meri. Ye to do din jindagani - You are not your body/ your body is not yours, so don't call it mine. Life is just two days long. – Kabir

March 28, 2013

I brought Madhukar to the dentist for his annual checkup. Nowadays he gets very nervous as soon as I take him to the doctor. He runs to the door to leave. But today he remained calm which put me at ease. That ease didn't last long when I heard the dentist, "Jyoti, you have to brush his teeth from now on. Madhukar is not brushing his teeth properly and his dental hygiene is not good". I bit my tongue while mentally adding yet another task to my already long list of everyday duties. That night I took him near the bathroom sink and told him to open his mouth. Like a stubborn child he clenched his jaw. I silently squeezed the toothpaste on his brush, hoping it would give him some motivation. But nothing registered. Again I asked him to open, but his jaw was still tight, and lips sealed. I tried to coax him and had him sit on the chair. Got a pot as a spittoon. Finally after a long time persuading him, he allowed me to brush his teeth. We both were very tired with this new task, which took almost 45 minutes. With a sigh he said out of the blue, "Jyoti, for no reason you have taken this extra burden on you."

I was shocked. His rare words pleased me immensely. He does surprise me sometimes with a sensible statement and makes me question the doctor's diagnosis about his illness. I helped him to sit on the toilet and left the nook to give him privacy. I pretended to wipe the sink and kept fiddling around, sneakily keeping one eye on him. I could see he just came out without wiping himself after he had his bowel movement. Without a word, I put the disposable gloves on and took him back to wipe him clean. I kept washing my hands with soap over and over again, turning into Lady Macbeth.

From then on, that too became my unwanted mission. I didn't like that at all. It felt filthy. But I felt sorry for him. Maybe it was my Karma. His hygiene was very important. Next day, we were almost finished with our dinner. Right then he had sudden gush of loose movement, effect of his Namenda. We couldn't even reach to the bathroom. It dripped all over the carpet on the way. I tried to clean him, but it was no use. So finally, I stripped him in the shower and bathed him again. I put on his pajamas even though it was early, in order to save me extra work later. I just didn't have any energy left to dress him now and undress him again at bedtime. I didn't do this lovingly at all. That feeling of resentment threw the dirt of guilt on me. I came back to my unfinished dinner. But the food was no longer appealing. Out of nowhere, Swami Jyotirmayananda's lecture resonated in my ears. We were attending a retreat in Chinmaya mission in Dallas.

'A young lad has fallen in love with a young maiden. Day and night, he only thinks of her. He has fixated on her beauty, the Mohini Astra. But remember, our body is constantly changing. Our youthful form will soon wilt into wrinkles. We are composed of many substances such as blood, bone, urine, and stool, etc. which is very dirty and not so appealing to us. We don't consider that beautiful. Suppose that young girl vomits. Then we could collect the filth in a bucket and show it to the lad, telling him, "This is also part of that beautiful girl whom you were dreaming about. I guarantee you he would run away and never look back. So Shankaracharya says, don't concentrate on your looks. The real you are the one who keeps your body alive. Worship that reality. the shakti, instead. Worship Govinda! He is your only savior, the one who is always constant.'

All the audience laughed at that. Later Madhukar and I read 'Bhaj Govindam' many times. He used to sing that bhajan. But I never really gave much thought to it then. After all those years, today the first time I understood the true meaning of Swamiji's sermon and what Shankara was saying.

***

She caught herself singing in the car when she dropped him at the day care center. She had only a few free hours as usual. 'Funny', she thought, 'the water in the pool seemed warmer and gentler today'. After a quick shower she headed for the parking lot and scanned the agenda for her chores. Groceries first, then stop at the optician to fix his glasses, go to the bank, get gas, call Dr. Nair. Reviewing the list made her dizzy. She concentrated on her breathing while the wheels began to roll. The sky was unusually blue today, she noticed. The fall colors were blazing! Borderland Park walks were their favorite in this season. For the last two weeks she had wanted to go there, but chores blocked her road. Without her notice, her thoughts steered the car towards the park. The green card for free senior parking was hanging on the windshield. They had applied for it as soon as they moved to this area, but little did she know that it would not be used for very long. The brittle sound of the dry leaves made a nice rhythm as she started walking down the road to her favorite spot. The rock was patiently waiting for her on the water bank.

Rocky terrain of her barren desire
She sows the seeds in her mind,
longing for warmth.
Suddenly the sky is thick with clouds.
The memories showered.
Gently sprouts the joy.
Shoots continue to burst out of the soil,
and she finds herself again.

She missed Madhukar so dearly. It was two years ago she was there with him, before the illness started. They had packed takeout subs and gone to watch the sunset. She thrust aside all the past memories and settled down quietly on the rock.

The sky and the horizon were melting into union into the lake. All the rocks and pebbles had found their firm abode in the water. She could almost hear the pine needles gently dropping down to join them. The orange and yellow leaves were surrendering into the lake. But the water stood still. It was not bothered by the chaos of the debris, nor did it become murky. The water was clear crystal. It allowed her to see the bottom of the lake. Her mind dissolved in that clarity and finally the true Dhyana, meditation happened in that magical tranquility.

***

March 28, 2013

I straightened the window curtain aside to see outside. John from next door was already on his morning jog. "Good morning, John." My raised voice did not wake Madhukar from his sleep. I went close to him and softly stirred him. Sometimes he gets up too quickly he loses his balance. I measured his sugar while he was still in bed. "Let's go to the bathroom."

A gentle reminder. I noticed he was disoriented. And became very shaky which becomes very difficult for me to handle him. I had to put a belt on him; only then could I take his adult diaper off. He got very stiff and refused to sit on the toilet. My thoughts started flowing. When the girls were little, I used to do the same exact routine, but with joy and adoration for their angelic gestures. Everything was cute about them. I would praise baby Chitru for doing su-su when I heard the tinkle of water coming from her tiny body. Of course, I was very young then, and they were my babies. Now doing the same thing for my fully-grown husband, my stamina has been exhausted. Poor thing, he is clueless. How can I blame him for my weak body? I try to keep him alert.

"I am putting toothpaste on your brush. Now I am washing your face."

"What am I going to do with the brush? Why do I have to do this?" His same old complaints harmonize with my daily instructions. I turn the shower on and signal to him, "Let's give your body a good scrub."

"That means you are going to take my clothes off. Never! I don't like to be naked." He repeats the same mantra while I start chanting my morning prayers in Sanskrit, hoping he will join in. He used to be a Sanskrit scholar. I struggle with his clothes in the midst of his nonstop grumbling. His essential dignity still exists deep down. I want to value his feelings the best I can. So I wrap the towel around him. Hot water is flowing. He just stands there, blankly looking at the cascade of water. I pull him into the shower. "Brahma murari triputantkari," I start the morning chants purposely to divert him. He used to sing that while taking his shower every morning. But today it doesn't reach him. I start rubbing Yardley's lavender soap on him. Maybe its therapeutic aroma or maybe the warm water sooths him a little. He becomes steady and calm. Next the difficult task of drying him completely, especially behind his ears which he doesn't like. Maybe the touch of the towel bothers him. I put him on the chair covering him again with his towel. Now I turn into a skilled navhi, a barber. To avoid skin cuts, I bought an electric shaver. I dab a few drops of Old Spice on his cheeks. I wonder if its fragrance brings some familiarity to him. He becomes very relaxed.

"Now how about a kiss for a tip?" Today to my surprise like a baby he puckers his lips towards me.

Following the podiatrist's strict instructions, I check all over his body for any open cuts and then start applying the special body cream on him. Dust anti-fungal powder inside his socks, and with a lot of struggle put the socks on his feet. Now one by one all the armor - the undergarments, the shirt, trousers, and then the sweater goes on his body.

Last task is to put the hearing aids on. I always have to remember to charge the batteries overnight. If they are not properly placed, there is a constant humming sound which is very annoying. In the beginning, I didn't know that could happen. Then he would get very agitated, not able to explain that it was bothering him, and he would have a temper tantrum. Over weeks of practice I figured it out finally.

Now the groom is ready, but what about the bride? I realize I am drenched as a side effect of his shower. I come to the kitchen and get busy. He follows me impatiently and starts pacing. I know he's hungry, so I start cooking his oatmeal over the stove. Suddenly he stands right behind me like a child holding on to mother's apron. I almost stumble over him. I struggle to keep myself calm.

"Raja, why don't you sit at the table?" I point him to the chair, but he doesn't move. He becomes more restless than normal. There is no rhyme or reason. Now abnormal has become the norm. "Don't make waves. Keep the same routine every day. Changes make the patient more confused," Natalie, our support group's director consistently tells her.

So to make him calm, I put his morning favorite Hariprasad Chourasia's flute on. Then the same old breakfast of old-fashioned oatmeal with milk, wild blueberries, seven almonds, and some walnuts which are good for the brain, and last comes the cinnamon. Hot pot of tea with freshly grated ginger. Stevia for his diabetes. Finally we begin our kingly breakfast. Despite all the things being served to him, his voice was harsh. His shouting filled the room.

"Jyoti, where is my medicine? Did you add stevia to my tea? How many almonds did you give me?"

"I have been doing it without a miss for the last 46 years." His ungratefulness makes me forget reality for a moment and my voice rises with irritation. He doesn't see any of the breakfast I laid before him. In his daze he gets up and shuffles towards the living room. I follow him and coaxingly bring him back to the table.

"Look how beautiful this spring is. It is giving us such positive energy. The frozen earth is welcoming the warm sunshine. Look at the birds at the birdfeeder, they have come back. The seeds in it are almost at the bottom, but they don't complain; they know Jyoti will refill it soon." My same everyday humdrum attempt to get him back. After breakfast, I do the same old drill again. Take the belt off, unzip him, put him on the toilet. The pain in my wrist is the same as I put his shoes on. I pack his lunchbox and write a note to his nurse, explaining his sugar level this morning. I should really xerox these notes.

Madhukar's favorite poem by Vinda Karandikar starts echoing in my ears…*Sakalpasun ratriparyant tech te ani tech te. Kakupasun Tajmahal, sagalikade tech hal. From morning through the night it is the same thing again and again. The same pea soup and same rubbery chicken...from the diner to the Taj Mahal it is the same story ...*

The ceiling fan is going around and round. Same as my endless endeavor of keeping my voice cheerful and calm. I keep him stable on the chair and get myself ready. Put his jacket and then mine on. Turn the alarm off from the night watch and turn it on again before we step out. How many rules and systems to follow? The community we live in is very safe, but Madhukar stubbornly insisted to install the alarm system as soon as we moved here. I didn't realize it then but in retrospect I think his ailment must have started then. One of the signs of Alzheimer's is a feeling of insecurity. I hold his hand and help him down the stairs. Push the button to open the garage door. Why can't they make a magical button to open the mind's secret door to happiness whenever one feels like?

"Today, you will get to do lots of interesting activities. I want you to follow the teacher's instructions fully so you will have fun." I secure him with a seatbelt. I have been doing this for the last whole year, yet still he reminds me as usual, "Jyoti, help me with the belt." That was our unwritten rule, never to leave the garage until you put the seatbelt on. I am so thankful to that seatbelt which saved Madhukar during his car accident in the past.

"We are going to the jail?" his everyday question resonates.
"All the staff there is so caring. They love you."

I ignore his remarks and assure him with my persistent response same as every day. But he doesn't budge and is crabbily protesting all the way to the center. As soon as we reach the parking lot, however, without any complaints he opens the car door. Doesn't even wait for me and walks inside.

Inside the center, the news and events of the day were being discussed. The activity director was reading a newspaper loudly to the group of special needs people in a circle. Madhukar was hesitant at the threshold. He forgot that I was with him. "Have a successful day today. I will be back at 3." I murmur in his ears. I had heard that greeting the first time in Frankfurt, Germany at my hotel as a wakeup call. I like the idea of starting somebody's day with such a positive greeting. I used to tell him the same when he would go to the office. I knew I will be doing the same drill in the afternoon when I bring him home and same again at night. Bill Murray in Groundhog Day lives the same day over and over again. The thought of following the same circus makes me tired already, and it is only nine in the morning. The news on the radio depresses me and my hand automatically goes to the CD player. Kishori's melodious singing is at my service. It soothes me; letting me float with her morning ragas. Don't know where the seven minutes flew by. I am at the health club and start changing in my cubby only to find out that in my morning rush I forgot my swimsuit. Frustrated, I start blaming myself for being so forgetful.

Today I really couldn't afford to lose the time. Chitra was taking me out for lunch. Mother and daughter's special time for bonding! I go back to my car grumbling, my jaw so tight all the laughter yoga in the car burned in anger. *Chakrvyuh* of annoyance surrounds me and I miss the exit to our home. Another stupidity on my part.

"If you miss the exit on the highway, you have to take a long turn to get back on the right road. Same is true of human beings. If you waste one life, you have to go through 84 million births to be human again." Swami Jyotirmayananda's words resonated in my ears.

Now I had wasted those valuable 20 minutes going back and forth. I am cursing under my breath while putting my bathing suit on in a hurry and finally I am in the pool. The little waves invite me with open arms, and I am one with the water. I am lost in the sound of the rhythm of my dancing body! I am at peace; I float and do my final meditation in the water. I pray to Goddess Maha Laxmi, '*I know you are taking care of Madhukar and protecting him. Let me serve my dear Madhukar with all the joy, peace and love; thank you for giving me the strength, wisdom and courage!*'

The tears add salt to the pool's water. The notion jabs me like a thorn that the sorrow has flooded over the joy and now all that's left is only a feeling of duty towards Madhukar. What happened to that Pativrata, the loving wife? What happened to that loving husband? Quickly ignoring my inquiries, I busy myself with my final stretching in the water. I can't digest the poison of this reality. I determinedly take the same vow over and over again, 'I will serve my darling husband with all my love.'

When I open my eyes, I see a woman walk on the pool deck. She looks like an angel because her white robe is flapping like wings. She steps into the water and comes straight toward me. She smiles gently and says hello. I return her greetings. Her smile assures my soul. Somehow, I feel very comfortable in this stranger's company. "How is your husband?" she inquires. I am a little taken aback, realizing that we must have met before. But I am not ready to show my lack of memory. We talk more. She tells me about her mother's dementia. I quietly ask her, "When was the last time we met?"

"Oh, in September," she answers. I am still not ready to admit not remembering that meeting. We chat more. I see my friend Kathy. She teaches swimming at the pool; she swims towards us and says hello to this woman. They exchange warm smiles. I ask the woman if she is here for swimming lessons from Kathy? She says no and smiles again. "Jyoti, you did not recognize her, she is my mother!" Kathy smiles back to me. I am relieved to solve the mystery about this woman and finally surrender to my honesty. I confess, "When I met you in September, you were sitting on the deck fully dressed. I am so sorry that I did not recognize you in your bathing suit and your cap."

We continue with our chit chat; she gives me a lot of good advice; I was right about her being my angel today. I confessed to her my failure to serve Madhukar with joy. I tell her, "Lots of times I feel that I am only doing my duty now." I told her what I prayed to the Goddess. She said, "All that is fine but add one more to the list for the Goddess. Ask her to give you serenity."

I sheepishly admit, "You, my angel of today, have given it to me." I leave the pool smiling.

***

I am on my way to enter my painting into an exhibit. But when I get to the gallery, I am told that the wire behind my painting was not proper according to their rules. I missed not having Madhukar by my side. He would have instantly repaired it. As soon as my paintings were finished, he was always eager to frame them and make them ready for display. *Gone are those days,* the harsh reality hangs over me. Soon, I need to bring him back from the day care. So the wiring will be added to tomorrow's list. I turn my car around. Just then I saw the Fresh Catch fish market in the strip mall. I usually don't go by there. The thought of fresh fish for dinner was quite deliciously tempting. I looked at the clock; it was almost 2:40 p.m. So I decided to stop for a quick catch. But then I saw a gas station with a lower price than where I normally go to fill up my car. Of course, every penny counts, the childhood saving habit never goes away. I was in the wrong lane, so efficiently I switched the lane to enter the gas station. I am expert at changing myself into an *Ashatbhuja.* In truth it was very much against to my yoga and Zen philosophy. No multi-tasking. But with all the chores I have to take care of in only 12 hours… My ears were engaged in *NPR's 'Fresh Air'* with Terry Gross. I missed the curve in my haste, and the wheels went up over the garden's bricks edge and got stuck in the muck. Alas, there was no Kaikeyi at my side to help me in this battle. I must admit that I become agitated sometimes and have temper tantrums like her. *"Jyoti pay total attention to what you are doing,"* Dada's words roared in my ears.

The clock starts running faster and competes with me. I am going to be late for Madhukar. The thought of him becoming anxious starts defeating me. By Murphy's Law, I had forgotten to charge my cell phone; I am not used to using it except for emergency. The battery was dead, so I couldn't call the center. I stood at the corner and abandoning all my inhibitions started my Macarena dance. Moving hands in the air to get attention from passing cars. But everybody was speeding by in their own hurry. Then one kind soul stopped and got out of the car, and before I could tell him my difficulty, he picked up the front of my car with his mighty arms and the right wheel got free. I didn't have *Tapsharya*, the power to give him a boon. I was overwhelmed by his kind help. Thought I would show my appreciation for his great service, by giving him some Bakshis. I opened my purse, took some twenty-dollar bills out, and looked up extending my hand - but he was already back in his car and zooming away. He didn't linger even for a moment for a reward. He didn't even allow me to thank him. I shouted loudly, "I owe you a big one! How can I ever thank you? I will pay it forward. I promise." My shouting was muffled by the traffic's racket.

'Karmanye Vadhikarasya Ma Faleshu Kadachan'-Your right is to perform your work, but never to the results. Never be motivated by expectation of the fruits of your actions.' He must have read the Gita. He was my angel that day. My mind humbly bowed down to his feet.

***

Day by day, Madhukar was losing his ability to do simple things. He had stopped putting the seatbelt on all by himself a long time ago. Now he was having difficulty getting in and out of the car. She had to lift him to get him in. That put lot of pressure on her and it aggravated her lower back. It was even more hard to get him out of the car. She had to coax him for a long time before he could cooperate and do the action. He was getting very unpredictable.

They were on their way to his doctor. Madhukar was in the passenger seat. Out of nowhere and without any warning, he opened the car door and was about to step out into the middle of the highway! Luckily, the seatbelt was still fastened around him. Her car was at high speed, 65 miles per hour, as were other passing cars. Her heart skipped a few beats knowing that he could have been crushed to death by the other cars. "Shut that door right away," she shouted at him as if his life depended on it. He was frightened and started shaking violently. He was not in the least aware of having done anything wrong. She could not stop the car abruptly. She slowed down a little bit but the cars behind her kept speeding. She was afraid for his life. She kept her left hand on the steering wheel and reached over him. With all her might she strained her right hand to close the door. She knew it was only a temporarily fix. The light signaled that the door was still open. In the next moment she pulled the car to the side of the road and stopped it. She was utterly shaken by the incident. He looked like a wilted leaf by her shouting.

She realized her mistake. *I should not have screamed like that at him.* She felt terribly guilty. She was so ashamed of her rage that she could not speak for a moment. Avoiding the speeding cars, carefully looking and making sure it was safe, tremblingly she got out. She went to the other side and opened his door. Rubbed his back lovingly. It calmed him down a bit. Before she could change her mind, without a word, she held on to his upper arm and pulled him out of the car and put him in the backseat. The locks on the rear doors were childproof. He started yelling but she didn't budge. She made her ears deaf and her mind hard as a rock. His safety was important than anything in the world. That is where he would be sitting from now on.

After they returned home, she could see he was very tired. So she made him sit on the sofa with his red shawl. Then she started stroking his head gently, humming a lullaby. His eyes started closing like a sleepy baby. Before she knew he was fast asleep. She also was fatigued by the incident. She laid down on the floor near him. She desperately needed the rest. Rain tapping on a sky light above. His snoring a dissonant rhythm. The ceiling fan gurgling. She forced herself to do Shavasan in spite of the cramps in her back. Her hot water bag was the only comfort she had in that moment.

***

October 5, 2013

Dawn's beautiful pink, orange rays peep through the curtain of the window and gently rested on her eyelids. She stirs from her good night's sleep - a rare occurrence! What a lovely way to wake up. She ignores the fast-ticking hands of the clock. Her morning is going unusually smoothly. She is almost done feeding him breakfast. His restlessness in the chair indicates the signal. She is becoming quite expert in reading his body language now, like the mother of a newborn baby. She helps him to stand and rushes him towards the bathroom. She had hoped his Namenda medicine's side effect was going down, but no such luck. It's too late. His diaper is already dirty, and he is completely covered in it. She starts cleaning him. She noticed she was holding her breath…

She starts chanting "Bhaj Govindam" in her mind while remembering Swamiji's teachings. Focus your attention on the real soul and not on the external body. She chuckles to herself mockingly - maybe with this ordeal she would witness the real Atman!

The stinky smell has filled the bathroom. Her fury's disgusting odor spreads along with it. She becomes ashamed of herself. Why can't I get used to it? He can't be blamed. He is beyond all awareness. She finishes cleaning him, forcing herself to hide behind a cloak of numbness.

Finally he is at the daycare and she is on her way to the pool. This time the clock makes her angry for her tardiness. Punctual Jyoti is gone, and her mind is still hovering in the morning's stench like a fly over muck. She is really disappointed with herself. How can she be still lingering in that stench?

She was relieved to reach the Holiday Inn. It was very crowded. So many women. Some were scurrying around carrying flowers in their hands. Others had very unusual things like bare branches, big tropical leaves, fruits, etc. What was going on? Maybe a flower exhibition? They had always gone to see the Art in Bloom exhibit at the MFA in Boston. Today the same flowers built a thorny fence of time around her. She couldn't spare that extra hour for leisure. Still, while going through the corridors, she stole a glance at the unusual flower arrangements. They were out of the box. Her mind's honeybee got locked in those flowers.

She too had always tried to use something different than normal in her flower arrangements. She flung away the time belt that constricted her neck. Her feet began roaming the rooms. Some of the flower arrangements were adorned with tomato stems, some with weeping willows droopy branches, some with only the flower's stamens, or only the veins from a big leaf! Every part of the plant was there. She always used big clusters of ginger roots, shiny purple eggplants, strawberries chopped with the green stem peeking out. But she wouldn't have dreamed of using what these women had. She was getting late for swimming, but she was floating on every single flower arrangement. Suddenly tears started flowing from her eyes. They are not sad tears; they are pearls laden with the joyous floral perfume. "Your exhibition is a beautiful invention," she says to the director of the exhibition. She does namaskar to her and thanks her again and again for giving her this extraordinary *Anubhuti,* experience.

Create art from the scraps of ordinary things. She breathed this mantra always. She was glad she was among her wild peers, free-spirited nomads. She had found Georgia O'Keefe many years ago when she was browsing through the books in Decatur's Library. Georgia O'Keefe was also traveling on the road less traveled. Instantly, the same as Eklavya's devotion to Drona, she became Georgia's devotee. With her unbound feistiness of an artist's tendency, Jyoti always felt that she was living on a lonely island. Today all the flowers gave her a blissful fragrance of moonshine to her thirsty Chataki[30] soul. Her lost smile shined like dewdrops. In the middle of winter, spring blossomed all over her body, and her desolate mind lingered in the oasis.

Enchanting Mexican music is playing in the corridors as she is on her way back to the parking lot. Without her noticing it her feet begin to pick up the beat. She dances as if nobody is watching her. Her contented mind is still trapped in the flowers. She sniffs the air. The earth is carrying Atma Sugandha, the aromatic scent of the soul, towards the sky.

Late afternoon sunlight pulls her into the backyard.
Way up in the sky an airplane hovering.
Gentle cool breeze goosebumps on her wrinkled skin.
The leaves of the tall oak tree shuffle into the wind song.

Little bells of the wind chime happily join their game.

Raven's sharp boasting screeches the atmosphere like nails on the blackboard.   The monstrous truck moans and groans with its changing gears on the road uphill.
While traffic the highway resonates like ocean waves.
Just then neighbor's house alarm sirens, but she mutes her mind to its loud shrills.

---

[30]Chatak is a bird in Indian mythology that waits for rains to quench its thirst.

Her favorite warm autumn. Its shimmering golden rays locks her in a magical moment.

***

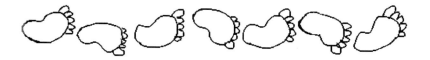

Sammohāt smṛiti-vibhramaḥ smṛiti-bhranśhād buddhi- nāśhāt praṇaśhyati - Anger leads to clouding of judgment, which results in bewilderment of the memory. When the memory is bewildered, the intellect gets destroyed. When the intellect is destroyed, one is ruined. – Bhagavad Gita

October 10, 2013

While the snow is still lacing the earth, a cold war between the winter and spring, a hole is drilled into a sugar maple's trunk. Sap starts dripping. The bucket is hanging just below to catch it and then that sap is transformed into a sugary maple syrup. *Daivi shakti, primordial cosmic energy,* is hiding within us like the syrup hides in the maple tree. In time of crisis and torments, the injured mind starts oozing sorrow. It appears to be a wound, but it is really a dripping of that cosmic energy in us. This is what she imagined. Like in a hive full of bee stings there is hidden honey. The double-edged sword of Alzheimer's was wounding them both.

Dr. Nair wanted to monitor if Madhukar's disease has crossed to the next stage. It has been more than a year since he saw Madhukar. Even though she was not a doctor, she could have easily guessed by Madhukar's deterioration that his disease has indeed progressed into the next stage. She fretted to take him for another long visit to doctor's office.

"Mrs. Joshi, Madhukar is not safe to be in the house anymore and neither are you safe taking care of him all by yourself. He might become violent. It is best to move him to a nursing home as soon as possible." Dr. Nair warned firmly to her and left the consulting room. She took him out of the consulting room. One case was done. "Next," the nurse called. An elderly woman escorted by a young girl passed them on the way.

The bitter truth she already knew became even worse when Madhukar didn't react to Dr. Nair's verdict at all. She was shocked that he remained calm without any reaction not uttering a single word. His silence screamed into her mind. *Who is he, an alien? Definitely not my lifelong mate.* Suddenly Madhukar became a stranger to her. When they were newlyweds, it was a romantic challenge to unfold all the facets of his unknown personality.

But now witnessing his unknown persona, she crumpled onto the bench in the waiting room. Bleakness covered her mind. The slamming of windowpanes awakened her back to reality. Outside, dark rainclouds burst into torrents. Furious tree branches pranced wildly in the gusts. The whole premises were being crushed by the storm surge, just as she and Madhukar were thrown about by the cyclone of Alzheimer's. Her mind was thrashing itself with one harsh query, "How can I send him to a nursing home???"

A flash of memory jolted. A man whom people called, '*Kadak Lakshmi-* fierce Avatar of Kali'. He was always dressed in a long skirt. He would start dancing fiercely on the street, in the loud beatings of the drums. His net of long hair wavering back and forth. Then in the middle of his dance he would thrash himself with a whip. All the kids in the neighborhood would run to watch him as soon as they hear the loud drums. She would to be terrified while watching his thrashing. She would be trembling with one excruciating thought - how could he tolerate such a pain? After all these years today she understood and felt his pain.

She was hoping that Madhukar would be an exception to all the research and doctors' predictions. But the last few months all her strength was absorbed by his inflamed symptoms. He was already at level three, out of five, when he was diagnosed. The bitter truth mocked. She would feel his hand slipping from her grip and watch helplessly as he fell down the cliff's edge.

Home or Nursing home? Her foot is caught between these two boulders. "*Jyoti, I am worried about you. I know you would take good care of your husband. But who would care for you? You need to be your own caretaker.*" Dr. Rosenthal's warning echoed loudly in her mind, and her determination to keep Madhukar with her evaporated. There was no choice but to give him up.

A depressing nursing home could never replace their beautiful Norton home. She dedicated herself to his tender loving care. How can that be swapped for indifferent employees? Anxiety pierced her lovesick heart. Her usual courage disappeared. Her willpower was diminished. She wanted to jump out of her skin. She managed to drive back home. She helped his tired body to settle down for a nap in the bed. She closed the door and ran to the living room. She flung herself on the sofa and began to weep hysterically.

The sturdy walls of her house were heartbroken by her wailing. They had never known this grieving sound. All they had heard previously were beautiful soothing melodies or her husband's thunderous laughter. They were shaken by her new Avatar.

'*Karu det shrungar sakhyano. Jiwantpani mi sati jatase*'- *Let me adorn myself for my beloved for the last time. I am a Sati while still alive.*'

Far away in the distance a train was doing its chugchug. Its whistle tugged her mind back in time to 1967, in their first flat in Dombivali. The full moon was peeking through the tree branch lattice. Her sleepy eyelids linger beyond awareness. Adoringly she held on to their first honeymoon, her mind dawdling in the hive of sweet memories.

***

He was away on a business trip and the girls were at college. I had always hated being home alone. I woke up in the middle of the night. A big meringue moon started pouring a sugary beam through the window, and I wished my Raja was with me to share this sight. I stood near the window, dissolving myself in that sweetness. Suddenly I heard gentle footsteps and felt someone else's presence in the room. I turned and saw Madhukar standing close to me, admiring the full moon. In my right mind I knew he was out of town. But I didn't give more thought to it and together we kept soaking in the moonshine.

I woke up the next morning to the phone ringing. It was Madhukar.

"Raja, where were you last night?" I asked.
"I was with you Jyoti, looking at the moon." He answered as a matter of fact.
I told him the whole incident in one breath. We both were so grateful to the *Great Almighty* for that sublime experience.

We were on our second trip to Scotland. We preferred to stay in B&B's rather than fancy, impersonal hotels. That way one gets a local touch. The house that we stayed in was a beautiful English Tudor. The owner, Suzan, gave us a little extra special treatment because she thought we were honeymooners! We both laughed and told her that we were twenty-two years married old couple.

Where have these twenty years gone?
I don't remember the Jyoti I was before I met you.
We've only just begun the journey of our seven lives together.
When did we get entwined so tenderly?
It is impossible to undo the tangles of 22 years.
I wake up every morning listening to your steady snoring.
At the breakfast table, we jokingly exchange, 'Did you have a good morning?'
On our walks, without a word spoken, I hear the rhythm of your heart.
Our shoulders rubbing unintentionally send a sweet surge all over my body.
When someone asked me a question, and you answered them instead of me,
the barometer of my anger would go up until you swallowed your words.
Still, I would never trade all this for a million-dollar lottery.
Is this what they call aged wine?

***

October 31, 2013

Anita was talking to me after a long time. Our heart-to-heart conversation began. Madhukar's illness, his suffering made her sad.

"Jyoti, why do you have to go through this horrible circumstance? Out of all the people, why God is punishing you?" she could hear Anita's sobbing.

"This is our *praktan*, fate. We are all born, carrying a sack of karma on our back. If your sack is full of rags, make a warm quilt. If your sack is heavy with precious gems, share them with others. Anita, I do see many jewels peeping through the rags in my sack," I assured her calmly.

Madhukar and I had woven a warm comforter from our beautiful loving threads of friendship. But now the blanket is tattered. All that remains are a few silky strands. When will they break? Until then I will not give up my *jidha* -strength. I have to go on, like the jute rope that does not lose its twist even when thrown into the fire.

Every day I am trying very hard to detach inch by inch from him.
Everybody's Karma is different at the end. Nobody really belongs to you after all.
After our marriage, our minds melted into one.
But now I would have to learn how to live on my own.
If only I could shed my love for him like a snake shades its skin, painlessly.
…Maybe to see him suffer is my fate.
Madhukar's disease is not just sucking his life but mine too.
Why is this happening?
Did I do something wrong in the past?

***

My thoughts wandered nonstop until I stumbled upon an incident …
Autumn was just about to be overcome by the harsher winter. The nights were cold and the ground was getting hard. A little baby

mouse looking for warmth settled down in our garage. I was annoyed by the sight of droppings everywhere.

Every time I tried to set a trap my own fingers would be caught. I went to Home Depot and the salesman came to my rescue. He showed me a new product, a paper so sticky that once the mouse stepped on it, it would be unable to escape. Much simpler than a trap. I was reluctantly sold on the idea. At night, though unwilling, I placed some cheese on the paper. I was racked with guilt. It was not even dawn when I ran downstairs to the garage. The mission was successful. But what I saw horrifyingly defeated me. Only one mouse leg was stuck on the paper. The poor mouse had gnawed its own leg off to save itself! I screamed. I had thought that I would catch the mouse alive and drop it in the woods behind our house. To make it suffer in such a horrible way was not my intention at all. But it was too late. My selfishness crippled this poor creature. Now reminiscing on this event, I think perhaps this is my atonement for that sin. Now just like that poor mouse I will have to gnaw my heart out to get free from this sorrow.

***

May 2, 2013

"Nobody else can do what you have done to take care of Madhukar. Jyoti, how do you do this?" Meena had asked her the other day.

"It's simple. How could I not do it? I am madly in love with him."

This morning Jyoti had a tough time with Madhukar. She just could not move his rigid body out of the car at the day care center. He would not cooperate. All her love could not carry his weight. Then she saw a nurse's assistance who worked there and yelled feebly for help. Together they were finally able to get him out.

She was momentarily relieved but the thought of doing the same at home worried her. Luckily, after expressing her concern to the social worker at the center, she found out that there was a bus service, for a fee. The bus driver would help Madhukar into and out of his seat. That very afternoon Madhukar came home by the bus. She saw the driver lifted Madhukar gently to get down. He held Madhukar's hand and again made sure he could climb the garage stairs. She was hoping that Madhukar would get used to this routine from now on.

She knew she would never be able to pay back the driver's kindness with any materialistic objects. Still she offered the driver a generous tip, but he refused with a smile.

"Please wait for a moment," she ran in the kitchen. Came back and stuff his hands with some fruits, candies and cookies-whatever she could find and muttered "One for the road."

Madhukar was having a hard time walking to the bathroom. His eyes were not focused, and he would lose his balance. Following the occupational therapist's advice, she bought red bed sheets. Red color is the only color these patients see any more for the most part. His dinner plate and coffee mug were also replaced with red ones. Dada's red shawl covered his sofa. Still, keeping an eye on him and protecting him was getting harder day by day, even with the gait belt. She knew the day would come when she would have to give his charge to somebody else. She would have to call the agency to start another caregiver for the two evening hours. Getting him ready for bed was exhausting. Finally, he was asleep. She had to pull her strength to climb the stairs upstairs. She sat staring at the computer... *The blaze of Alzheimer's was engulfing the house. They were both charred in its flames. Suddenly a Phoenix flies out of the fire. Its wings spread high in divine inspiration. It returned to her... she began to write of her beloved's sacrifice. What a ransomed price they both are paying. Would there be light at the other end of this tunnel of his suffering?*

***

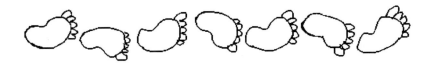

A birthday is just another mirage on the path of life. - Unknown

October 7, 2013

The bright moon stirred her sleep. Dawn was about to melt into full sunshine; she should really get up. But instead she pulled the quilt over her head. She remembered that it was *Vat Purnima*, the full moon dedicated to Savitri. Did Savitri really get her husband back from Yama, the god of death? She had never believed those stories from her childhood, but Madhukar's illness had made her weak, and now she felt only if she could follow in Savitri's footsteps. She wanted another baraat with her beloved on this Purnima night, his smile by her side, his zest for life. But he was in the no moon phase.

"Happy Birthday to my Raja, today is your special day." I landed a gentle kiss on his cheeks while waking him up. "Madhukar, it's your birthday, so I'm going to do aarti to you in the evening when the girls come," I the queen announced cheerfully.

"Good morning and happy birthday, Dr. J," said his favorite lady in waiting, Silvia. "I am going to dress him in style for this special occasion," Silvia told me as she went to his closet and I took him to the bathroom. He just stood there, staring at the mirror. I became a fly on the wall.

He looks in the mirror.
But the face on the other side is not recognizable!
Who is that person?
Just a blank stare.
Scrawny face covered in the web of premature wrinkles.
Who is he?
Who is he?

Uncertainty is shining through the mirror.
Maybe it is the wrong mirror?
Slack muscles have removed the smile from the face.
Who is he?
Who is he?
Don't know him at all!
The room is flooded with the photos.
I think I know that person in the photos.
I feel close to him. Did I have a twin?
Maybe he does not live here anymore, where did he go?
How this proper stranger allowed in the mirror?
Uninvited, unwanted!
Must find that old mirror.
Must find the keys to answer these questions.
The tongue swallows all the words.
Only loud muteness is ruling.

Silvia rescued me from bathroom duty. I was happy that he didn't see my tears. The pact that I had made with myself when he was diagnosed with Alzheimer's was to never cry in front of him. The 75th birthday is a very big celebration in Indian culture. But he was beyond a party. I knew this was going to be his last birthday in our Norton home. The bitter truth wasn't going to stop me celebrating full blast. Regardless of his blood sugar, I decided to cook a feast suitable for my Raja. Breakfast was served – Ras Malai, and banana muffins made especially for him by his daughter Chitra.

"If you are happy and you know it, clap your hands," words sleep through my mouth, on our way to the day care. To my heart delight, I heard a soft clap, from the back seat. The sound of his claps-*Nadbramha* kept vibrating in my heart.

His 75th birthday celebration began in full force since yesterday. I had cooked all his favorite food. Without a word he gobbled up all the dinner, stuffed sole with goat cheese, spinach stuffed mushrooms, spring salad and snap peas.

Even though he could not really handle going out, today I made the decision to just go to the nearby Fresh Catch restaurant with the whole family. As soon as the food was served, he gulped it all. When his plate was empty, he got up abruptly from the chair. He kept looking back and forth to the exit door. It's time to go home! He was not going to wait for anybody to finish their food. I told the girls, "Please do not rush. Enjoy your dinner, I will take daddy home."

As we return, I lit the candle on the dining table at home and started chanting our evening prayers, *"Shubham karoti* ... Let the atmosphere be filled with blessings, let all the dark be destroyed by this light …"

He was standing very close to me, yet I felt very much alone. I laced my fingers into his and confessed, "On this day, I have no present for you except my unconditional love!"

I took shelter in our favorite *Marwa* Raag, perfect for dusk… *"Piya bin suni sej*… *Bed feels empty without my beloved*!"

It was only seven o'clock, but he was already dozing must be all that food. I prepared him for the night and settled him in bed, tucking the two pillows on each side as a barricade so he wouldn't fall. I knew his leg would still cross over this barrier in the middle of the night and I would be awakened. Our large king size bed and I sleep almost on the edge, but I don't mind it because his being next to me is my ultimate comfort.

I should really look into the hospital bed that Silvia had suggested. I wondered why the doctor had not told me of such a simple solution. Pushing the button would work like magic, bringing him upright from a sleeping position.

***

The day goes by without a single word from him. But at night in his sleep I hear some gibberish that quenches my thirsty ears. In the middle of the night, he gets restless. My hand gently touches his scalp to make sure he does not have hypoglycemia. I rub his back so he could fall asleep while my own rest is shoved away. The sleepless night will add to my backache tomorrow. But I will firmly ignore it and convince myself again to keep every pain in my body in control, otherwise who would look after him?

This same pattern continued in the following days and weeks. There is only one solution – to sleep upstairs in the guest room. But how can I leave him alone downstairs? The last 46 years we shared the same bed. For the few days I slept on the living room couch, so I would hear him, just in case. But the couch was narrow, and it felt like I was in a train sleeping car. Now I know why prisoners are deprived of sleep, so they can easily be made to confess. But I never felt that I was in jail. I was a captive all right, but only to his love. He is incarcerated by this horrible disease.

***

Next day after dinner she took him for a walk after tying his gait belt on, a new addition to his attire. She met Donna on the road. When Donna heard her sleep problems, she gave Jyoti her baby monitor which would help Jyoti to hear Madhukar wherever she would sleep.

That night Jyoti resolutely made the decision. After getting him ready for bed, she scurried upstairs to the guest bedroom before she could change her mind. She slowly gathered her magical tools to fall asleep: Tiger balm for pain, towel to cover her head, socks for her cold feet, hot water bag for her back, melatonin pill, a book, and glasses.

But there's no sleep-in sight. "*Piya bin suni sej*". She has never slept alone until today. As a child she slept between her parents. After marriage, she was with her husband. When the four of them would watch TV at night, she would tell them to turn it off and go to bed because of the 'late hour'. But the real reason was that she didn't want to go upstairs alone. She hated to sleep alone. Finally, she falls asleep all alone in the guest room.

***

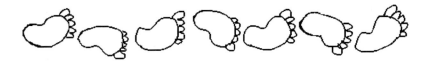

***Good night Irene, Good night Irene...I'll see you in my dreams.
- Huddie 'Lead Belly' Ledbetter***

January 3, 2014

He hurriedly followed her in the kitchen like a child trails his mother. She distracted him by pointing at the little toy bullock cart on her kitchen counter. In the past he would immediately start playing with it, his hands moving the cart back and forth. But now he can't even do that. He is sinking further into infancy. The TV was blasting. He yawned, eyes heavy with sleep. "Come on, you need to go to bed!" She said lovingly to him as if he were baby Jeevan. After tucking him gently in the bed, she whispered in his ears,

"Do you know how much I love you? More than all the buds that have bloomed. More than all the snowflakes that have fallen. More than all the stars in the night sky. It would be impossible to measure the length of my love."

One of Harry Belafonte's songs came to her mind. He had introduced Belafonte to her when they were newlyweds. She started singing it as a lullaby to him, "Good night Irene, good night Irene."

Lo and behold. All his vows of silence washed away. He started humming the last line with her, and in the next second, he was fast asleep.

From now on, it became her routine to sing that song at bedtime. He would go without uttering a single word all day, but every night she would hear him singing very clearly the last line of the song as a promise to meet her in his dream. She eagerly looked forward to their duet. She made sure all the caregivers would always recite that song for him.

***

The nor'easter was in full force for the last two days. After hearing the weather forecast, she made sure to stock her refrigerator fully. The power went out, but luckily, she had gathered the emergency flashlights and batteries. She had always loved the snow-covered earth. Sipping hot chocolate, her nose touching the glass window like a little girl. She would be mesmerized by the shiny white reflections of moonlight on snow. But now that same Jyoti couldn't find that beauty or peace in that same whiteness. The roads were blocked, and nobody could go out. His day care center was closed. She felt imprisoned in the frozen wasteland of Alzheimer's. She was locked in with him alone for two unbearable days without the caregivers' assistance.

Cabin fever set in, 48 hours without anybody to talk to. She kept the TV on for him, but its constant noise gave her a throbbing headache. She was completely stressed out. It was the same feeling she had after giving birth to Swati, with nobody around to help during the daytime.

Finally, the third day arrived with bright sunshine and the phone rang with welcome news.

The roads were clear, and his caregiver was on the way. She was so happy to hear the announcement that she hung near the front door waiting for the bell to ring. At last the caregiver arrived, but it was Lisa. His usual caregiver Melisa was sick, so they sent somebody brand new. Never mind, Jyoti was so happy to have another speaking person in the house that she did not mind explaining Madhukar's whole elaborate routine to her. She asked Lisa to help Madhukar with his daily stroll in the house as she hurriedly rushed to her respite, her computer!

She had not written anything for the last two days. She took a deep breath and started putting together all the scattered pages of her disrupted life. Her ears hoping to hear his footsteps, but a heavy silence that made her uneasy. She called down, "Lisa, could you please sing something to him while walking? He likes that. It really helps him."

Lisa sheepishly said, "I only know two songs."
"Oh! Good, then sing those two," Jyoti gently requested.

"Good night Irene, good night Irene..."

Lisa's melodious voice caressed Jyoti's weary mind. How did Lisa know that was our special song?

"In the middle of a tempest, Lisa, you my special angel, came to my relief today!" Jyoti went down the stairs hurriedly to hug Lisa with joy.

***

September 27, 2013

My girls warned me not to go alone in search of a nursing home, but they only had only weekends to themselves while juggling their jobs and other responsibilities. So why add another demand to their already busy life?

I ignored their warnings. Searching for a nursing home was against my wishes, but still I started hunting for a good place for Madhukar on my own. First, I went to nearby ones, then a little further, but nowhere satisfied me. I even went to see some assisted-living facilities, where both of us could stay together. Every time I came home empty-handed and more depressed.

Some of the places were not kept well at all; as soon as I entered, the odor of urine made me nauseous. A lack of cleanliness, cheap and bland food, dark rooms, shabby furniture in need of repair, patients wailing in their beds. Outside at the nurses' center I would see the caregivers and other staff with a coffee mug in their hand chatting away, seemingly aloof to the patients' calls. My guts would be twisted, and I would start running as fast as I could to my car wiping my tears... away from those nerve-racking places called "nursing" homes! I knew that could be my reality. But I would not think even in my dreams to send my beloved to this kind of facility. I was determined to keep him home with me forever.

My fatigued body was no longer able to care for him. The thought terrified me. "You must send him to a nursing home," Dr. Nair's warning echoed in my ears. I forgot to breathe for a moment when I finally confronted the ugly truth carved in stone that I could not erase, that Dr. Nair was right. So were Swati and Chitra when they begged her, "Ai, we need you to be around for Jeevan's future wedding." I remembered how much I missed Aai-Dada when they were not present in person to give their blessings at the wedding of Chitra and Mark. Who knows about the future, but right now I needed to surrender to the present.

***

"Aai, from now on I forbid you to go to look for nursing homes alone." Chitra's firm command was echoing in my ears. I got an appointment to visit Epoch right near me. So Chitra and I went, hoping that this place would be satisfactory, as at least it was in walking distance.

'Joy and Peace', Namaste[31] - was written underneath the white paper dove hanging on the door to the Alzheimer's ward. I was comforted a little by this coincidence. Our own front door at home was adorned with Picasso's dove representing world peace. All my letters are signed with 'Love, Peace and Joy!' Soft music was playing in the room, small flag-shaped paper banners gently swaying with the rhythm. Nature scenes were scrolling silently on the large tv on the wall.

The wrinkles on the patients' faces carried the burden of many years. Behind their Alzheimer's masks, sitting silently in wheelchairs with blank eyes. They did not notice us! A nurse was painting bright nail polish on the old woman's fingers in bright red color... Red color shrilled an alarm. My mind revolted," *No! No! My Raja has not reached their level yet; he is definitely NOT like these motionless patients!!!*"

---

[31] Namaste is a greeting in Indian culture, welcoming others and saluting their inner light.

"I will *not* send your father here! Did you look at that woman, how she is lost? Daddy does not belong here." My eyes welled over even as I firmly whispered to Chitra.

"*Mamuli*, our Daddy *does* look like them, staring at the ceiling, lost somewhere far away, depressed and scared, not knowing where he is! His whole world has shrunk down to the space around his easy chair," Chitra reminded me gently, while rubbing my back with motherly love.

The little flicker of *Jyoti* became a blaze, and my peace blackened. I grabbed Chit's hand firmly and fled hurriedly from that *Namaste* room.

"You can put down a deposit now, so his name will go on a waiting list. When there is a vacant bed, we will let you know," the secretary assured me.

The truth was a bitter pill to swallow. I could see there were plenty of patients waiting to leave their bed and exit forever. The nursing home was like a lion's den into which one entered but never left. Many days passed, and the secretary never even returned my phone calls.

We visited another local assisted living halfway between my house and Chit's house, which was very nice indeed. Unfortunately, they didn't have round-the-clock nursing care so they would need to call an ambulance for something as simple as a hypoglycemic reaction, which was not uncommon for a diabetic. I would also need to arrange for a visiting nurse for his insulin injections. Besides, there was no vacancy. In a way I was relieved since I didn't have to decide right away, so it bought me more time at home with him.

***

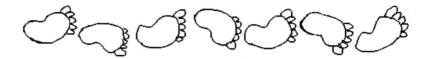

January 29, 2014

Orchards Nursing Home[32]

My torturous search to find the best nursing home was in full swing. One day my friend Ann-Carole suggested another nursing home, where her husband was staying. Even though it was far away, I considered visiting it. I had known Ann-Carole for a long time. If it was good enough for her husband, it must be okay. So, I was looking for directions on the computer and suddenly right there on cyberspace's magic screen another nursing home appeared, *Orchards Rehabilitation and Nursing Center.* I had heard about it before, but it was almost 15 miles away, so I had disregarded it at that time. Now, however, it suddenly seemed closer compared to the one that Ann-Carole mentioned.

Chitra and I went to explore the Orchards nursing home the very next day. As I parked the car, immediately the surrounding woods made me feel at ease. Orchards was owned by one family for the last 40 years. That alone was enough for me to realize their commitment. Still with a heavy heart I gathered my courage holding Chitra's hand and proceeded towards the entrance.

"Jyoti, this is going to be his second home. We will try our best for his comfort," was the guidance counselor Melanie's very first sentence to me. Her assurance helped me to find long lost peace as we entered their reception area.

She led us through the clean, shiny corridors with soft music quietly playing to a large dining room, decorated with round tables wrapped in red tablecloths and fresh flower centerpieces. There was also a small private room for families to dine in. A gentleman was playing

---

[32] Not the actual name.

on a grand piano where other residents were sitting quietly. They had a facility for pedicure/manicure, hair salon, and arts & crafts right on site, and the eye doctor and the dentist came monthly. There were two doctors who made rounds once a week, which meant no longer a need to drive to the medical center to get all his prescriptions. They had around the clock nurses on staff so Madhukar could get his daily insulin shot.

They had a special locked memory ward for dementia patients. The rooms were clean and well-equipped with decent furniture, fans, and air conditioners. All these luxuries came with a higher price, but I was determined to starve if I had to, to ensure a quality nursing home for Madhukar. Chitra and I were both very impressed by Orchards' caring staff.

The overall ambiance of the facility was peaceful, not depressing like all the nursing home that I had visited before. It felt like a four-star hotel, but of course Madhukar was not able to even notice it; this was all for my satisfaction only.

With our luck they had a room available for him.

"Please save that room for him," I told Melanie as I signed the deposit check and escaped from there before I could change my mind.

The next day I took him to the day care center and gave notice that he wouldn't be coming starting next week. Their social worker exploded a bomb on me, "Jyoti, that will be his end! Don't send him to the nursing home!" It crushed my serenity. It was the most difficult decision that I would have to take in my entire life.

***

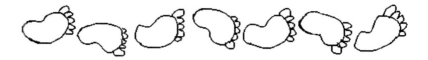

January 12, 2014

47 years ago, on this day, we tied the knot. All the years flew by with rainbow colors on my wings. Destiny hoots and drowns out the melody of wedding Shehnai[33]. The seven rounds we took around the holy fire, turned into an inferno... swallowing our very beings. Enchanted journey of seven steps has taken a wrong turn today. I would rather swallow a glass full of poison than be separated from you, my beloved.

Defying the frigid air, I went to the garden center to buy yellow roses that he used to buy for me always.

I started to set the dining table. Thorns from the long stem yellow roses in the center piece pierced my finger. Drop of red oozes out. My heartache is far redder than this drop. *'Don't allow the tempest from your heart to surface, keep moving forward'*... Aai's unspoken advice through her actions constantly resonates.

I put on my 'smiley face mask' to celebrate our anniversary.

Two golden candelabras stand next to the roses. The crystal chandelier from the ceiling sways gently in approval.

Dinner special is simmering on the stove: butter chicken, saffron biryani garnished with cashews and golden raisins, Navratan curry, raita, stuffed mushrooms with sunflower seeds. Swati brought tiramisu and, mango cheesecake, as if this were not enough, Chitra added additional desserts of chocolate mousse and pistachio *kulfi*... *a* feast appropriate for my *Raja*.

---

[33] Shehnai is a musical instrument often played at weddings as a tradition.

'*This is his last supper in this house.*' The chandelier dimmed for a second and froze in shock as I bit my tongue for allowing such a negative thought.

We sit down for dinner as I lit the candles on the table and chant prayers of thanks. After dinner, I honor him with Arti, the five-little *Diyas-ghee* lamps. Light glows on his face, but his eyes did not reflect light from the Diya.

Swati, Chitra, Mark, and Jeevan said their goodbyes and left. Like every night, I got him ready and tucked him in bed for the night, stroking him lovingly a little more than usual, lingering more than usual.

Then I rushed upstairs, repeating loudly, "*Forgive me my love, my hands are shackled by the cruel reality. It is not safe anymore for you to stay at home. So many times, you fell in the last few weeks. The other day, you bumped your head so hard on the floor, the wound in your head would not stop bleeding and then in panic had to call 911. My hands are no longer strong enough to pick you up.*"

The harsh reality kept ringing a bell all night… 'I will have to call Orchards nursing home tomorrow, to set the date for your departure.'

***

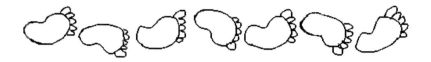

Two logs gently floating side by side in the ocean...one wave breaks them apart, and they never see each other again. - Poet G. D. Madgulakar, as translated from Marathi

February 6, 2014

She woke up in the morning, but her timid mind could not face the shiny rays of the morning sun. She just could not gather herself to tackle the world today. Finally, she put on all the armor to challenge the frigid air and started walking in the neighborhood. Her feet felt so heavy as if they were chained by iron shackles. The thought of packing his bag made her tremble. She moved around in a slow-motion film.

Ann-Carole was also taking a stroll, her straight necked body so erect that you would think she was in an army drill. Vision fixed far away, holding tight to the leash on her dog Freddy. One foot after another. Such determination...How does she do it? Nobody will ever suspect she had been scorched by caregiving for her husband, who passed away a year ago. Ann-Carole was unaware about Madhukar's new home.

"Hello Jyoti," Ann-Carole greeted her.

Just a nod of Jyoti's head... her unusual mute answer from quivering lips and teary eyes gave it all away.

"Jyoti, what's wrong?" Ann-Carole stopped right away, patting her gently.

"We are moving him tomorrow to Orchards nursing home. Will you please pray for him, Ann?"

"Of course, I will, you know that. I am always here for you. Tell me what I can do for you," Ann-Carole assured her.

That night when they went out for their stroll, she could not locate Venus. The breach between them was too wide. She looked at the North star for guidance, but it did not give any. She looked at the trees, they did not wave at her…the birds were already hiding…the clouds…they all turned away from her. She felt so alone.

***

The merciless Friday morning of February 7, 2014 arrived.

Both girls arrived before the scheduled time. Jyoti could clearly see Swati's stress, her unusual rush in getting things ready due to all the heartache she felt… her father was not going to be at home anymore. Jyoti caught Chitra wiping her eyes secretly as soon as she entered the house.

She was also not herself… Jyoti prayed silently to her Goddess, 'you are the only one who can look after him now,' then she called her two brothers in India for their blessings. She avoided giving Madhukar a spoon full of homemade yogurt… it is an Indian tradition that when someone leaves for a journey, the lady of the house feeds homemade yogurt to the traveler in hopes that the sweet taste would encourage the traveler to return back soon.

She held on to his soft hand tightly in the car as the familiar surroundings of the neighborhood swiftly vanishing behind them. "I will never leave you, my love, remember how you used to go on business trips? Well that's how it is!" She continued the same dialog repeatedly, trying to convince her own mind. Sadness crowded her mind, as if she were trying to find the way out of a thorny jungle. It was a relief when she realized that Swati had parked in the Orchards lot.

He was received with a warm welcome smile by some of the staff at the front… as soon as they entered, everything started moving as a factory assembly line. She and her daughters had sorted out their own jobs.

Swati took charge of her father, making sure he is settled down in his new room. She fed him lunch from Orchards' kitchen. Chitra started unpacking his suitcase, hanging his clothes in the closet, mounting some family photos on the wall. Keeping his favorite books of Asimov's science fiction and Lincoln's biography on his bedside stand. They knew that those books were there just a stage prop. Jyoti was assigned to talk to the staff. *'Nobody would be able to take care of him as lovingly as me'*... The thought kept pounding her heart bleed. She had concluded reluctantly that no matter how many instructions she would give about his care giving, all of them were just hired help.

"We are ready for you, Mrs. Joshi," the chief of staff Kent, his arms resting on his waist, announced with smile. Deja Vu... His shiny dark purple black skin, white of the eyes ... pulled her all the way back to her youth. Vithoba, the *avatar* of Lord Vishnu, same cockleshell eyes, same obsidian skin. Vithoba's temple was on the street where she grew up, and before every exam she would go there for his blessings. She felt some relief because of this similarity and pretended Vithoba had come to save her. Sending Madhukar to this strange place was the toughest test she had ever faced in her life. When she heard that Kent was originally from Guyana, Africa, she immediately requested, "I know your people value the closeness of family, same as we Indians do. Kent, please consider my husband as your uncle and take care of him with tender love."

Nancy, the dietician, asked Jyoti lots of questions about Madhukar's eating habits. Then the director of the home, Kathy, her assistant Jill, the social worker Melanie, and Madhukar's daily personal caregiver Mary came by. Jyoti felt smothered by all their questions.

"This is Linda," Kent introduced the main nurse in the ward to her. She was so surprised by hearing the familiar name. Her mind flew 44 years back when they bought their very first house in Framingham. Next day the doorbell rang, and a couple came to meet them with warm banana bread in hand. They were their neighbors David and Linda! They had three boys. Linda always wanted a girl, so when she heard about Jyoti and Madhukar's daughter Swati she was thrilled. Linda offered to house-sit to hand out candies to Halloween goblins since they had a Diwali function that same night.

Another time, they were away from home when a snowstorm hit. Madhukar was worried that he wouldn't be able to get into the garage since the driveway would be packed with snow. Lo and behold, as they approached the house, they saw to their surprise that the driveway was completely clean. Some angel had come and plowed it overnight. Next day they found that angel was David. He often came to their rescue to help fix things in the house over the years. When Madhukar would thank him, David's usual answer would be, "Oh, don't thank me because I get to experiment and learn to fix things that I have never done before!"

They became close. Linda took Jyoti under her wing. When Linda's mother Myra came for a visit and heard that her daughter's neighbors were from India, she was delighted. Myra strongly believed that in her last life she was Indian. She followed Indian philosophy deeply.

Later, wherever Jyoti and Madhukar had moved, one of their neighbors would always be named either Linda or David. Their Norton home was no exception – there was a Linda right next door to their condo. Now in this new home for Madhukar, his nurse was Linda, it was a good sign. "What more can I ask for?" Jyoti was overwhelmed with relief; her anxiety faded a little bit.

…But she could not let herself linger in the past and get distracted from all the questions she wanted to ask this Linda about Madhukar's medical care. Kent started reading the 5 pages of information on Madhukar's daily routine that Jyoti had written so carefully. His medicines, his diabetic diet, his daily habits, his likes and dislikes - the list went on and on. She was drained after giving a full report of her last four to five years of her tender loving care of her husband. "Can I send my wife to you to learn?" he asked her, amused.

"Kent, I have cut my heart open and given it to you. Please take extra good care of him, I beg you, please," her eyes welled. Taking care of Madhukar, she never once thought it was strenuous work. But now when she saw all the details of all her daily chores suddenly, she felt weak.

***

By now it was almost three o'clock in the afternoon. It was time to leave him at his new home. She could not face the separation. She felt that Madhukar knew deep down what was happening. Ever since they entered his room, frown wrinkles had had appeared on his forehead and his face was pouty. Did he recognize the new surrounding? Did he feel scared? Abandoned? She would never know the true answers.

She hugged him again and again, lingered on the threshold and finally pushed herself out of the room. The girls and she had made a pact beforehand that no matter what, they would not shed a tear in front of him! They would cry only in private. As soon as she reached the parking lot, she lost all her control, wiping tears with the back of her wrist, she told Swati to start the car so she wouldn't run back to him.

Not a single sound except puttering of the car. She was afraid if she attempted to utter anything it would only come out as sobs. When this horrible disease took over to Madhukar, she never blamed destiny or asked why? How? But today she howled at her beloved goddess Mahalaxmi, 'Why are you punishing him? Why couldn't you choose me instead?' The thought of losing him completely even though he was alive, blasted a huge hole in her mind as she entered the house.

The house had always felt full in spite of the fragments of his vanishing personality. But now as she entered the house it felt vacant like her mind. She started drowning in that vacuum. She forced Chitra to return to her own home, as their fatigued bodies clung to each other in goodbyes. After Chitra left, she and Swati collapsed on the king size bed into a deep nap from the sheer emotional exhaustion until the phone startled her. She pushed the button on answering machine, "Hi Aaji, I know today Ajoba is in his new home, so you are sad, so this is for you. Kissy mmwaa." Jeevan's sweet voice lifted her spirit a little bit. She was grateful to have such a darling grandson, apple of her eye. He had tied Ajoba around his little pinky! His wish would be Madhukar's command! Jeevan worshipped Ajoba. She was the one would take care of Jeevan, giving him baths, feeding him, bringing him from school, but every time Jeevan entered the house, his first inquiry was always, "Where is Ajoba?"

"You little rascal, I am standing in front of you, at least ask me how I am!" Aaji would shower him kisses and hugs in mock anger.

Jeevan often came to sleep over, always begging to sleep in between them and ask Ajoba to, "sing your song *Jo Jo Jo re*"-a lullaby. Madhukar might not have done that for his daughters but he would do anything for this little prince. As his illness took over all that pampering disappeared. The loving Ajoba turned into a grouchy man. He could not tolerate Jeevan tagging behind him. The father who never once raised his hand to his daughters now spanked his grandson twice without the least provocation. Jeevan's lips would quiver while trying to understand why Ajoba was so angry at him. The thought that Jeevan might only remember this cruel Ajoba frightened Jyoti. She decided to make sure Madhukar's loving persona would be always alive in Jeevan's mind. She started telling him stories of their playtimes, showing him old videos and pictures of baby Jeevan with affectionate Ajoba. She planned to take him to Ajoba's new home to make sure he understood that Ajoba was still very much part of the family.

The darkness of her mind reflected the darkening evening outside. Swati and she hurried back to the nursing home to see him. He looked tired. She fed him his supper tenderly. Then the caregiver got him ready for bed under her guidance. She wanted so much to tuck him into the soft white cotton ironed bed sheet. Determinedly she locked her hands and stood aside, resisting the temptation. The nurse gave him an insulin shot. From now on Jyoti was released from her daily duties of nursing him, but she hardly felt free. Would they take good care of him? Would they pay attention to his needs? What if? What then?? Thousands of questions built an iron wall of prison trapping her inside it forever.

He fell asleep instantly. With a heavy heart she entrusted him to Melanie's hands, and holding on to Swati, walked quietly out of the room. She felt the pain of a young mother who gives away her newborn baby for adoption. Madhukar was very much there, alive in body yet so far away, beyond reach as if there were seven oceans dividing them.

Mother and daughter reached home and ate dinner in unusual silence without the usual chit chat. She felt again the abnormal fatigue she had never experienced before. Slumber swallowed her like a tidal wave, and she slept as if she had never slept before!

In the morning she told Swati firmly, "Please don't worry about me. I will have to learn to live alone! Don't forget I am my Mother's daughter. Same genes you girls are carrying also. No matter what, never give up! I have learned that from your father. Do you remember, when he had a car accident and could not walk for a long time? He never stopped trying until he was able to walk, ride a bike and finally climb mountains again. Remember his exuberance and strong convictions! Please return to your job, your home, your life. Your cat Keshoba must be waiting impatiently for you!"

***

Next day she woke up early, very eager to go see him right away. She went to the living room to open the curtain and stopped short … On the wall was hanging his most favorite, painting by her, 'Abhisarika'[34].

She was transformed into that woman… January 1977, their 10th anniversary. Creativity came dancing to her that morning. There was no canvas in the house. She went crazy looking for something she could paint on …She found a white cheesecloth. too tender to paint on but that didn't stop her muse. Putting bold brush strokes on that surface, she lost herself until Abhisarika came alive. Madhukar came home from the office that evening and he just stood in front of that painting speechless…but the twinkle in his eyes and profound joy on his face told her all. No need of words! She was pleased that he liked her present on their special day! Without ado he started on a project, forgetting about dinner all together until he

---

[34] A woman who is eager to meet her lover.

was able to put a frame around that painting. He never allowed her to sell it ...Suddenly that painting became a splinter in her eye. "What is this painting doing here?" her mind demanded.

She draped the painting in a soft comforter, putting it carefully on the back seat, her car raced to his nursing home. *'If only I could swaddle him in my love and carry him around everywhere, I go.'*

The custodian was hammering a nail on the wall, but she felt it on her heart. No, I will not become sad in front of Madhukar, she reminded herself again, and she crammed her emotions in the same comforter. Madhukar raises his hand to her; that made her happy. She caressed his soft hand - with his magic touch, the soft quilt of all the memories unfolded.

***

June 1969

I had accepted the new career of wife and mother to a newborn full heartedly. Yet, I wondered if I would ever dig my way out of the piles of dirty diapers. Doing the household chores and preparing gourmet dishes, etc., was no longer enough for me and this created a lot of turmoil. I realized that only when I nurtured my passion and followed my dreams, I would be able to be a good mother to Swati. I decided to get back into my art. I entered in the exhibition at the University of Illinois, and to my surprise won first prize. I entered many exhibitions after that, and rarely missed getting first prize. Every time that happened, Madhukar would embarrass me by bragging about my success to our friends.

My photo, along with a one-page interview about me, appeared in the local paper after one such an exhibition. Poor Madhukar, because of him I came to this country, but he merited only a one-line mention at the bottom! He could not have cared less about the slight but instead showed off his wife's fame to everybody who entered our apartment.

I was amused by the articles effect because people would point at me and whisper. I was being recognized on the streets of Decatur now! Not just as that 'exotic' Indian woman in a sari but as an accomplished artist. My muse started blooming, nurtured by my Raja's whole-hearted support. Of course, my paintings started orbiting around one topic, 'Mother and Child.'

***

Madhukar hung all my paintings on the wall of the Framingham Public Library the day before my very first solo exhibition. So many rounds of carefully carrying all my paintings from the car into the library.
My first one-woman event today. As the opening time approached, I became very nervous. I felt as if I would be naked in front of the viewers. Madhukar noticed my apprehension and exclaimed,

"Don't be silly. You are not introverted like me. You are always able to express your emotions freely like a butterfly. Today people are going to witness the real you, all the rainbow colors of your artistic mind. They will taste the sublime in your art. Don't be afraid. Come on, wear the beautiful sari that I bought for this special occasion. Get ready, remember the reporter from the Middlesex Newspaper is coming to interview you."

Buoyed by his pep talk, I quickly got ready while remembering his sweet promise during our first night to give his heartfelt support to my art. Instantly he became my muse, my Raja, king, my savior.

That exhibition was very much admired by the public and became a successful foundation for my future shows. A reporter from the Middlesex News came to our home afterwards and asked me very straightforward questions. The next day there was a full-page article from him in the paper. Remembering my parents' teaching, I tried to humbly brush it off and continue working hard. I knew I was only holding the brush; the real artist channeling all the paintings through my hands was someone else.

My confidence grew stronger and wherever I moved, from Massachusetts to Texas, I entered competitions and gave solo exhibitions, earning critical acclaim. I was truly blessed.

The last exhibition I took part in was in 2012 at Harvard University. There was a Q & A session after the opening. The auditorium was fully packed. Ever since his illness took over, I had avoided these kinds of crowds which made Madhukar very restless and agitated. I knew that stress was not healthy for him and that he would lose his patience. Still, remembering how much he had appreciated my art, the girls and I decided to bring him along anyways. It was extremely difficult to take care of him while attending to my paintings, but we took that risk because it was essential for my soul that he be there. Swati and Chitra tended to his needs while I went on stage.

"Where does your creativity originate from?" somebody in the audience asked.

All the artists on the panel remained hesitant. I saw Madhukar sitting in the auditorium between my girls. I forgot about his confusion and illness, and my mind thrived to see him there. His presence gave me tremendous courage. Pushing my stage fright away, I rose to answer.

The disease consumed his speech and intellect, but I still could feel his mute support. I saw a little spark of admiration in his eyes, shining out through his vanishing persona, and it gave me my confidence back. I nodded him silently and gave my answer to the question.

"When I am holding a brush, I witness the creator in me who takes over and I as Jyoti no longer remains. Creativity originates only from the Creator." The audience applauded loudly in response.

He sat still the entire time without trying to get up to leave the room. His being there was an exponentially higher reward than exhibiting at Harvard University. *He is the man standing behind my successful art.*

***

The next few days did not flow as easily as she had wanted. The separation between them was impossible to endure.

She did not straighten the wrinkles out of her unmade bed.
Her favorite morning raga Lalit did not play as usual on the CD.
Breakfast dishes remained grubby in the sink.
She neglected herself along with the house.
She had been his shadow for the past five years.
Now the distance of 15 miles felt like fifteen thousand.
She was not there to rub his back in the bathroom if he became fidgety.
She wouldn't be applying cream while gently giving him a massage after the shower.
She wouldn't change his position after sitting too long in his chair.
She wouldn't wipe his drools throughout the day.
She wouldn't be lighting the candle on their dinner table for the evening prayers.
No more lullabies or goodnight kisses.

It was getting late. She finally turned off the bedside lamp. She lay there without getting a wink of sleep, face down in her bed lifelessly. The darkness of the room seeped into her mind. The red numbers on the clock, as if hot coals in the fireplace, started scorching her mind.

***

The calendar kept unfolding each day making it too long. She still could not find her song. She felt as if she was being torn apart from him. Every day after feeding him lunch, she returns alone to her home which was no longer his home too. She would tell him, "Ok, I will come back after I finish grocery shopping, I am going to the library," giving him excuses but never saying the word goodbye to him.

She kept reminding herself again and again on her way back from Orchards. Her thoughts, her mind, her heart is hinged on him. Unseen to others he is still by my side with every step I take. Maybe the silk shawl of our intimacy is ragged, but its soft touch is the same.

'I am a free woman,' at least that was her belief but without her knowing it she became a captive in his fading kingdom. Her mind started hammering her only one thought: I must detach myself from him. Our paths are no longer the same.

As she pushed the garage opener from her car, *the garage door moaned,*
"Would you please oil my hinges?"
As she climbed the stairs to the house, the tangled cobwebs on the ceiling whispered,
"Please set us free."
The knotted strands of her hair grumbled, "now at last give us a shampoo."
As she put the bag of groceries on the kitchen counter, the dabba full of spices opened its lid, *"would you please cook something delicious just for yourself?"*

***

It has been almost a month. She pinched herself, because today the house did not seem to be empty without him. A carousel of thoughts went around and round, taunting. *He was not even here anymore. As soon as Alzheimer's branded him, he left you and went in an unknown world. You were in complete denial and kept holding on to his shadow.*

She wanted desperately to escape from her mind's accusations. Their happy life in the past lured her. They had just landed in America. Honeymoon was still lingering. But she knew she could not go back in time. It was like going after a mirage.

She could still smell his aftershave on the towel in the bathroom…The house was too silent; she was not accustomed being all alone in the house. She could not bear the separation. She longed for his return.

Determinedly she turned the shower on as if she could wash away all those memories. Perfume of Yardley soap mixed with the steaming hot water to soothe her body... and started pouring into a cascade of words...

Raja, I want you to be right here at this moment.
Dark clouds are gathering in the sky.
I started the car lost in my own thoughts.
The raindrops started tap dancing on the windshield.
At that very moment I wanted you right there,
your voice echoing as a drumbeat.
At the breakfast table when I cut your favorite fruit,
its vermilion color burst all over,
and I wished you were there by my side to savor the sweet mango.
You used to go for long walks, leaving me alone at the beach.
I wanted you to come back to me right away,
so we could jump in the waves together when the high tide returned.
Yesterday when watching a funny sitcom,
giggling all by myself,
I wanted you right next to me with the thunder of your laughter.
When our favorite Marwa drenches me in its sweet melody,
I want you to meet me at the crescendo.
Look, there is a cardinal at the birdfeeder with its mate.
I wish you would take flight right now towards me,
Showering me with your kisses.
I need you. I want you.
Right now. Right now.
Finally, after a long day, I rest my fatigued head on the pillow.
I need you right there next to me, to get lost in your embrace.
I need you then I need you now.
I will always long for you.

***

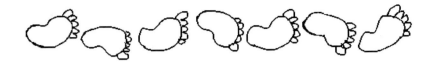

Be the change you wish to see in the world -- Mahatma Gandhi.

Constant streak of tears became my only make up for my eyes. I would be awakened in the middles of night to find my pillow soaking wet and catch myself sobbing uncontrollably. Charred by his absence, his love, my mind was parched and getting whipped by these wet lashes.

Every time I entered Madhukar's ward, I would see him sitting on a chair facing the TV, his eyes frozen on the show uncomprehendingly. Was he far away singing his own tune or sinking in the deep darkness? He reminded me of an old, wrinkled tortoise sitting motionlessly on a log. Sometimes when I walked with him, people would mistake him as my father. He had aged so quickly with the ravages of this disease.

Within few days, even though Orchards looked like a four-star hotel, I realized Madhukar was being neglected. He was eating fancy food, the room was modern and kept clean, still he was missing the detailed personal care altogether. I noticed that Marie, his care giver, did not even brush his teeth daily. I never heard her speaking to him kindly, I tried to talk to her, but she would not change. Her rudeness continued. This was unacceptable to me. At home he was cared for deeply. I always made sure his dignity was valued. If he was given tender loving care at home while I was the only caregiver, then why couldn't that happen with the army of caregivers?

The very first day I had taken him to Orchards, the social worker Melanie had warned me, "You will have to accept that nobody will be ever take care of him like you did. It might take 2-3 months for him and for you to get adjusted. Don't worry, but I want to assure you one very important thing, if you find something wrong, then report it to me immediately."

As I was leaving Orchards that afternoon, the turmoil in my mind blended with the outside storm. I was swept by tortured hopelessness. I made a horrible mistake sending my husband there. How can I mend it now?

The next day I went back in a bleak mood. Madhukar was sitting in the TV room with the other residents. I patted his shoulder and held his hand. "How are you Raja? Oh my god! What happened to you?" I wailed. His right cheek was bruised, and the right side of his face was black and blue up to the eye. "Did you fall down?" I kept asking him, forgetting he was not able to answer me. *I am his voice! I am his voice!* I stormed to the nurse's station in the corridor, trying to keep my voice low. Still the tigress in me, saw her cub harmed, took over and roared,

"How did he fall? How could you not watch him? You were supposed to keep him safe!"

The nurse told me aloofly, "Jyoti, he did not fall. Last night he was sitting next to Lisa, watching TV. Lisa hit him then."

"What was the supervisor doing? Am I paying such a high price for him to get injured?" I lost my composure. "Poor thing, he can't protect himself, and you can't do it either? Make sure that this will not happen ever again. Keep him away from Lisa and take good care of him."

I stomped into Kent's office crying. His room full of cheap aftershave gave me a sinus headache. I demanded an explanation from him, only to hear his false promise, "I will look into it." His kind resemblance to *Vithoba* vanished and he turned into a weasel. His teeth shined like hyena's crooked smile. I left his office with a throbbing anguish.

Every day I would find some new occurrence. The very first day, Madhukar's shoes, underwear, shirts, pants, pillow cover, and bed sheets were stamped with his name in permanent ink. Yet Nick, whose room was next to Madhukar's, was roaming the halls wearing Madhukar's blue shirt. I tried to ignore it. The other day when I walked in, the first thing I noticed was that Madhukar was wearing only one hearing aid; the other one was missing. His hearing aids were top of the line, very tiny but very expensive. Poor Madhukar would be more confused if he can't hear well. Nobody even noticed that he had lost it. Again, the same drill; I complained to Kent, he promised to replace it. It took them a month to get him another one, which was not the same quality. He already lost his slippers last week. Every day I would go home more and more depressed about sending him there.

***

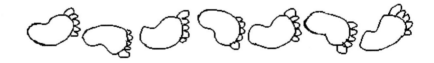

Problems are simply challenges waiting for solutions. The two are partners. Think positively that a solution will appear, and it will. – Unknown

April 8, 2014

She stirred in the middle of the night. He was sleeping right next to her in the bed. How is this possible? She jolted awake. She could not see his body but definitely felt his solid presence. The bed sheet was slowly moving up and down with the rhythm of his breathing. She was not imagining it. She could not touch his body, but she knew he was there. Was it an outer body experience? She wanted to keep him there forever. All night she laid still as a log, not even a slight move. Time stood still. It was like "The Twilight Zone." Oh, how she was suffering from their continuous separation. She wondered if he was also missing her, and that is why he came to visit her. 'I must ask him, but how? Silly me, if he could answer the mystery, then he would not be in the nursing home in the first place! Or maybe another miracle would happen, and he will speak to me today!' Entangled in the maze of her strange thoughts, she did not realize when she reached the Orchards parking lot.

Every time after leaving him there alone, Jyoti would be in excruciating agony, his gloomy face would cover her with sadness. Not only would she bring Madhukar home in her mind, but she also carried along all the other residents from his ward too. In a strange one-way communication with them she knew them all by now. She would toss and turn sleepless in her bed at night, hoping only for him to return to her like the other night, but the other unwanted residents would crowd in her mind instead.

She became attached to Orchards' surroundings; its walls begin to reassure her. When she visited, the other patients were the same as Madhukar, moving around endlessly without uttering a word, and silently staring at her. But she would try to understand them, coaxing them gently. As soon as she entered, she would start talking to them as if they could understand. Today was no different. As she entered through the locked door, she saw Roberta standing there clutching her two baby dolls, imagining that she had just delivered those twins. Georgia quietly sitting in her wheelchair kept a watchful eye on everyone. Grace was all dressed up, with gaudy makeup and bright red polish on her manicured fingers, in a hurry to go somewhere. She was constantly pacing back and forth. In the corner of the TV room, Marvin, 99 years old, was nonstop moaning, drooling, and speaking gibberish. Teresa was in the room next to Madhukar's. She was bedridden; her husband Ted was, as always, sitting at her bedside. Teresa's condition was the worst compared to all the others. She was losing the fight against cruel Alzheimer's. Six feet tall, blue-eyed Ted looked a lot younger than his 80 years, always joking, smiling, and facing the day ahead. Maybe because of their common bond of suffering with a spouse, Jyoti and Ted started exchanging little friendly chats. One day Jyoti saw him entering the ward a little late. She had never seen him walking with his head down, anxiety exploding all over his face. She tried to console him, "Don't worry, if you are late today, Teresa will understand."

"Jyoti, Teresa died yesterday," she heard, whispered through his quivering lips.

"Oh, I am so so sorry, I did not know," Jyoti started shaking, could hardly control her sobs. A week after that Roberta left this world after having a slight fever. Maya followed next. One after another, everybody was leaving to another world. Jyoti could not escape from this harsh pattern. Scary thoughts stormed through her. Large wide TV in the recreation room, beautiful flower arrangements in every corner, soft music in the background, nice rooms, delicious meals, all this was in a tunnel to nowhere. All the residents were waiting for their train of no return. When she brought Madhukar here six months ago, she did not even comprehend that someone else had gone to his final journey so Madhukar could gain the bed. This ruthless truth with its piercing claws started gnawing at her mind.

"Jyoti don't send him to the nursing home, that will be his end," said the social worker at his day care center, her bitter verdict cutting Jyoti like a sword.

***

I was shocked to see everybody was walking around with a mask on their face at Orchards. When I entered Madhukar's room, he was still in the bed on his side towards the wall. I think he heard my footsteps. Nowadays, this was his new way of protesting-turning away from me. I saw his mask when I went around to greet him. The nurse told me about widespread flu in the nursing home. I just stood there quietly hoping that he will be safe since he already had a flu shot. There was a calendar on the wall, Swati's birthday was marked on today's date. Did Madhukar write it? I was puzzled for a moment, then realized that I had brought that calendar from home with all the important dates marked on it.

He started pulling his mask away… at that very moment the past put another mask of a memory on my face.

April 8, 1969, Decatur

The sundown started some pain in my lower belly. We both have taken the prenatal classes to learn, how to take care of yourself and the baby, how to breath when the labor pain starts etc. I recognized the pattern of my pain. My bag was already packed. After an hour when the labor pain became unbearable following the doctor's orders, we headed to St. Mary's hospital. Fathers were not allowed in birthing room. All alone, I remained calm and prayed to my Goddess. I missed my *Aai* so imagined that she was right by my side. Because of the practice in the prenatal class, I was prepared. Within two hours, our daughter Swati was born.

The doctor put the crying baby on my stomach. Witnessing, experiencing this miracle of birth I was overcome with infinite gratitude for this baby, made from my own flesh and blood. The sky was too small to fit my love for her. Swati's two little dimples so visible even when she was not smiling, they possessed my whole universe. First time in life I utterly understand exactly what the element of motherhood was. Tuesday was a holy day of Goddess Mahalaxmi. It is believed that Laxmi enters at the dusk. Swati was born on Tuesday evening. I took it as a good omen.

Two days in the hospital ended quickly, admiring Swati's every single koo and kaa. Madhukar was driving us back to the home. Both of us had discussed and took the decision carefully not to invite my Aai for help. I had seen other parents who come to help for the childbirth, end up working hard. No maid or servants to wash the dishes, clean the house or do the laundry all the unending chores. Nowhere to go without a car. My mother did not speak English. The American lifestyle would make her a prisoner in our home, we definitely did not want that.

But right now, all that firm determination melted away and I longed to be near my mother. If only I was in Dadar right now? Bringing home, a baby would have been big gala celebration not just in our family but whole Narayan Niwas would take the active part in it. People would be stopping showering the new baby with gifts and blessings. I, the new mother would be pampered- resting day and night for first six weeks with delicious almond and ghee halwa, plus nurturing three meals and a massage every day for next three months… My daydreaming churned with the car's wheels.

As the car stopped in front of our building. I was fretted, devastated by the thought of entering to an empty apartment and begin to take care of this newborn all by myself. Nobody would be waiting to bless little baby Swati. I carried my little bundle of joy carefully to the third floor to our apartment. I was surprised to see a big poster on the door.

"Welcoming Home Baby Swati, we wish you all health."

The door opened from inside. Judy my next-door neighbor-my dear friend, was waiting in our apartment with open arms for Swati and me. The tears of bliss and humble gratitude started streaming down on my cheeks. Judy had filled the whole void of *Narayan Niwas*. She became my whole village.

Madhukar dashed in the bedroom and scurried back with covering his face with a mask and plastic gloves on his hands.

"Why are you wearing those?" baffled by his attire, I asked him.

"Don't you remember Jyoti, in the class they warned us that we must protect the baby from germs. That is why I am wearing this mask," he confided in me proudly.

"Dear husband, did you forget you are baby's father. She will not get sick by our germs. On the contrary she must get used it!" I laughingly tried to convince him. But at the same time, I was convinced that Swati and I are tied together with this absent-minded professor forever.

Later that week, Madhukar's boss Dr. Eicker, who was a psychologist, came to see the baby. On that day as he was leaving, he said,

"Jyoti don't forget to live your life also. Don't just concentrate in taking care of your baby all alone. Do keep her with the babysitter and go out often." Listening to his so-called advice, I was boggled. What does he mean by babysitter? I had never heard of that word before.

Swati would wake up in the middle of night for feeding. Deprived by sleep, I would be dragging myself the whole day walking like a zombie. I could not tell if my day started or ended. Holding Dr. Spock's book in my hands, I started learning the technique of motherhood. I was alone in the house with Swati. No adult to talk to, until Madhukar would return from work at 6 in the evening.

All the dirty diapers, sterilizing the milk bottles, cooking and other house chores, nobody to help me. I was not able to rest at all. I began to feel very depressed. And then suddenly Dr. Eicker's words came to my rescue. I became aware of its true meaning…

Now back in Orchards with Madhukar's confused expressions, I wondered if I could ever find Dr. Spock again for this grownup baby?

***

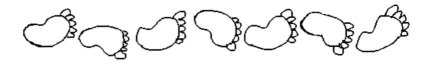

***We never know how high we are till we are called to rise -
Emily Dickinson***

After swimming, she returned hurriedly as usual to the Holiday Inn parking lot. Rain or shine, this was her routine for the last 7 years! It was already 10 o'clock in the morning. Since she has become a one band woman now, hundreds of tasks to accomplish!

The carefree days of childhood rolled in her mind like a classic movie reel. She would play with her friends after school and go to the Mumbai Chowpati (shoreline) for evening strolls. She later regretted that neither she nor anybody else swam in that beautiful Arabian Sea.

Her mother had enrolled her for swimming lessons at the Mahatma Gandhi Tank. On her very first day when she felt the lifeguard's hungry gaze all over her and other young girls in the pool, it disgusted her, and she refused to go back; her excuse being too bashful to wear a swimsuit. That was the end of her swimming until she came to America with her husband; only then did she learn swimming at the late age of 21. But ever since then she was a fish in the water!

Drenched in her thoughts, she came to the car. The sound of drums startled her. She was surprised to see a Barat, a wedding procession, in the far corner of the parking lot. Men and women draped in colorful Indian kurtas and saris were doing the rhythmic Garba dance with the colorful wooden *dandiya*.

The music brought a huge smile to her face and her car was automatically lured toward the Barat! She loved wedding ceremonies and could not remember the last time she had attended such a joyous occasion. Nowadays her social life had come to nil. Her body slowly started moving with the rhythm of the drums. The past began to dance with the present. The first time she danced Garba was at Sumati's wedding, her best friend from college. In America she had begged her husband to join her in taking ball dancing lessons. He went just to please her but was so stiff he would invariably step on her toes. Now her craving for dancing was doused with Zumba at the senior center.

The loud thumps drummed her back to reality. She rolled the car windows down and allowed the music to seep into her soul, feet gently tapping. A rainbow arc glided from the sky into a circle of bright vermilion, yellow, orange, and green saris! Riding on a white horse, the handsome groom suddenly appeared inside that orbit as if he were the Sun, the center of the bride's new universe. What a lovely sight! She quietly blessed the union of the newlyweds, 'Nanda Soukhybhare! May you live happily ever after!' She then left that enchanting moment to meet her own bridegroom, who was waiting all alone in the nursing home, garlanded with Alzheimer's.

***

She wished the calendar would forget to turn the months. But no such luck! 'He must be waiting for me impatiently like he used to at the daycare center', innocent hope sprouted. She knew that was not happening; on the contrary, the door of his mind was rapidly shutting. Never before had she felt so desperate like today. Her mind moaned, 'He is evaporating since he went to the nursing home.'

Still she followed her discipline, having become a robot. She would not miss a day of feeding him. Today was no different from other days, except she woke up feeling very restless. The horizon seemed bleak to her, with no muse to be found. The house felt more barren than ever without him. She was clutching a delicate strand made of her one and only desire, to find a remedy for his recovery. She was a fly caught in the spider's web, struggling to get out.

She felt she had become a machine that constantly churning. One of her favorite paintings from college days was 'Man, Time and Machine.' After so many years it still hung on her mind's wall. The machine took over the clock and turned the creator, the man himself into the machine, trapped by time. What an easy life it was then; she had not been enslaved by that clock; she had been carefree as a bird. Then where did the inspiration for that painting come to her from? Was it a little glimpse of her future life?

The police abruptly stopped the traffic and the train of her thoughts. She saw the ambulance by the side of the road and spotted the accident. As her habit, she sent healing prayers to the victim. She clutched the steering wheel tight and murmured under her breath, 'Oh no, this halt will upset my schedule, I can't afford that!' She noticed the huge boulder peeping out of the woods across. She had fondly observed that rock many times before, but today he appeared to be signaling her. Valiantly sitting on the earth but deeply rooted in her mind. She started pondering, 'how does he do it?'

She is flabbergasted by his firm attitude.
He watches with complete detachment,
as a blade of lush green grass flirts with wildflowers.
She had seen him once,
stark naked,
contemplating life in the middle of a bone-biting cold,
enduring layers of frozen ice.
Then she remembered the thrashing of heavy rain showers on his bare back,
The blistering rays of the sun.
He is always standing steadfast, stable and focused.
Cold, rain, sunshine, he does not care.
His silence confronts her demandingly,
'If a mere rock like myself can observing the world without pain,
then what is your problem?'

At last the police signals to the traffic and her car moves on, only after she promises the rock to follow his example and stay balanced. Today she understood why all the rocks under the trees in India, dipped with orange paint, are worshipped always.

***

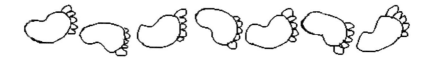

Keep your face always toward the sunshine and the shadows will fall behind you. – Walt Whitman

That same evening, she decided to go to the new art exhibit at Wheaton College. When they had first moved to Norton, she had immediately joined the Wheaton College programs. Madhukar and she used to attend every single exhibition. She was not able to do such a simple thing spontaneously now. After talking to the artist, she got inspired. Tomorrow was the monthly meeting at the local art club, which she had stopped going to in the last few years. So that became the next thing on her agenda.

As she was driving back home the sun was setting and the sky burst into beautiful vermilion, pink, and violet. They used to keep the camera on the back seat to indulge their common passion of capturing nature's treats. She wished the camera was still there. She did not remember when she last used it. She pulled her car near the side of the road.

"I think it pisses God off if you walk by the color purple in a field somewhere and don't notice it. People think pleasing God is all God cares about. But any fool living in the world can see it always trying to please us back." Alice Walker's words pounded in her ears.

'*How could I ever turn my back to nature's abundance?*' She moaned silently and started absorbing all that beauty. The dusk was generously pouring itself into her soul and brought her a deep joy that she had totally forgotten in the past few years. She hurriedly parked in the garage and ran upstairs, computer turned on, fingers moving fiercely with the brush from the graphic art app, her mind flying. She was pleased to see the sunset appearing on the screen. Nature was giving her all its beauty; it would be truly sinful if she ignored it.

***

Next morning dawned with a joyous mood. I cooked his favorite lunch and got ready to visit him earlier than usual. On the way I realized that I needed to print yesterday's painting so that I could enter the upcoming town exhibition. The wheels read my mind and turned towards to Staples. Seeing the long queue in the store, the worm wriggled impatiently. I took the number and sat in the chair to wait for my turn.

After a few minutes of dozing, my eyes opened to see a middle-aged couple standing in line. His hair was tied in a ponytail and hers was short, almost a crew cut. He gently touched his lips on his lady's neck, her smiles like a sweet dream. The lady took out a white shell from her pocket. He saw it and gave her a happy nod. No words were exchanged but their silence sang loudly.

Nanda Soukhybhare', the blessing flew out of my lips. The white seashell sunk deep into my mind. The vast ocean of memories rolling. Madhukar and I used to sit at the seashore for hours, without a word, just enjoying the waves and soft sand, collecting numerous shells. The big pink conch that Madhukar brought me from one of his trips, trumpeted in my ears. Our backyard and every corner of the house is a collection of the beautiful shells. I collected the canvas and rushed to my car in that mood of Abhisarika.

He was in his reclining chair, leg stretched, his vision blank without any spark. 'Who is this stranger? Does he feel the same about me? Doesn't matter,' I rebuked myself sharply. I recognize my beloved. That is enough for me.

"Hi Raja, I can see you are ready to go for a walk with me."

I gently coaxed him to stand and tied the gait belt around his waist so I could manage his balance. At the same time, I tightened my own lumbar belt not just around my paining lower back but to rein my mind in too. I kept my neck straight, and holding his hand, together we started our walk in the corridor, one step at a time. Finally, our feet found the same rhythm of trudging.

'Prison', he used to call the day care center.
Now he is locked behind the doors of the Alzheimer's ward,
not even aware of his confinement.
He is beyond locks and borders.
he is truly free.
I am finally living my life independently,
but this forced freedom feels like prison to me.
Life has become a circus in my tent with only.one pole,
Wearing a clown mask.
I am the roaring tigress,
and I am the ringmaster who controls the beast inside me,
always with a whip in hand.

***

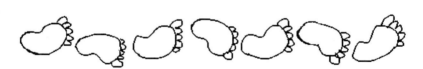

September 24, 2014, the first day of Navaratri

She had reluctantly accepted the reality in Orchards. Nobody could match the loving care of a wife to hired help. At least he was safe. Twenty-four hours on duty, the nurse was there to give him meds and the doctor came on his regular rounds.

She entered Madhukar's room, well aware of his declining health. The girls also observed this, but no one had the courage to discuss it openly. His walking completely came to a halt. Now his only mode of transportation was a wheelchair to be pushed back and forth in a cruel game of musical chairs from the bed to the bathroom, from the bathroom to the TV room easy chair, from the easy chair back to bed. About a month ago, his head dropped down suddenly. From then on, he stayed in the same position, no longer able to hold it up. It was hard to feed him; still she managed somehow.

"Let's get some vitamin D, soon these warm, sunny days will be history." After lunch, she pushed his wheelchair all the way outside.

The Indian summer was pleasant. She sat on the bench and turned his wheelchair towards her, taking his leg onto her lap and massaging it. He would have never allowed her to do such seva-service before, but now, neither could he protest nor complain about the cramps in his legs caused by sitting in the same position all day.

"Today is the first day of Navratri festival," she murmured to him. The famous Mahalakshmi temple in Mumbai appeared in her mind. Getting to ride in a taxi was her biggest lure to go to that temple with her Baba uncle. Inside the shrine, the shiny gold face of Mahalakshmi adorned with studded gems fascinated that eight-year-old girl. She could not remember exactly when Mahalakshmi's face began to be to carve into her heart. She started accompanying Dada while she was in college in time of Navaratri festival, and continued following the ritual every time she would visit her motherland. She could always feel the hidden *shakti*-super power in that temple.

After becoming a yoga practitioner, she got away from worshipping idols. But every time she would meditate, Mahalakshmi's face would appear in front of her. she became a devotee of the Goddess. She was confident that Mahalakshmi was constantly guiding her in Madhukar's sickness. Mahalakshmi's face would greet her with a smile every time she woke up in the morning or went to bed at night. Right now, sitting on that bench, the same thing happened. She continued her chanting,

"Ya devi serv bhuteshu Matr-rupen sansthita-you are a mother who resides in every living being."
Every time she started chanting prayers or mantras, he would utter a word or two, but that has stopped now. Caving in, she pushed the

wheelchair toward the door to take him in, but suddenly she stood still. She felt the presence of her goddess. She circled her hands around his neck like a garland and whispered lovingly into his ears,

"Raja, get ready for your final journey. This is the auspicious Navaratri muhurta - my Aai chose Navaratri to end her journey on this earth. I give you my consent to bid me goodbye. Please don't worry about the girls or me. You have taken such good care of all of us, by providing for us all of our lives. You kept us happy. You are a good soul mate, protector, provider, loving father, and husband. What more could I ask for? It is only in your hands to stop this suffering. You alone can do it and be one with God almighty."

She stopped trembling. Nobody would ever know how much strength she had to pull from every cell of her body to proclaim the harsh decision. She was certain, Mahalakshmi was behind this unusual courage. Today was the first time she left Orchards with dry eyes.

***

October 1, 2014

The next few days brought altogether a different scenario. He kept chewing food for a long time without actually swallowing it. He was forgetting how to swallow. Sometimes he would not even touch the food. His pattern of not eating took Jyoti's own appetite away. She was feeling guilty. Did he hear her request? Is that why he was on a 'hunger strike'? In the early stage of his illness, she had to hide food away from him. He would forget that he had just eaten lunch a few minutes ago and would immediately have a temper tantrum for lunch again. Whatever food he saw, he would grab and gobble it hungrily.

She had started using aroma therapy to relax him. They both were fond of *Mogara-Jasmine flowers.* One day she had just plucked a handful of Mogara flowers from her garden and held them out for him to smell. "Look, a gift from paradise," she showed him adoringly. Immediately he reached for it and put a handful of the flowers in his mouth. She was stunned by his action; never could she imagine that he will eat them. Before she could open his mouth, they were all disappeared. She let out a big sigh of relief that at least Mogara is not poisonous.

Another afternoon, she realized it was too quiet in the house, so she had gone looking for him. He was pacing back and forth, happily chewing something. There was no food around, she struggled to open his mouth. He was chewing tiny pebbles! Her collection of colored pebbles from all over the world that she kept in a glass bowl that once she made it in her ceramics class.

Her mind shouted at her, *'enough of all this Feng Shui and decoration! Make the house safe for your husband!'* She went all around the house like a hawk looking for hidden things that he could find to put it in his mouth.

***

October 5, 2014

Swati was at Orchards, trying to feed her father that morning. He could not respond to her at all. Swati called her mother in panic, "Aai, Daddy can't even open his mouth."

She had knowingly not told her daughters about his new phase. Sometimes he will open his mouth as if he wants the food. She would become hopeful that maybe his appetite is back but then he would chew the food without swallowing for a long time. Other times he would go without food for days. She could not endure how the disease was tossing him back and forth like a cat and mouse game. She consulted with his doctor and their discussion concluded that there was nothing they could offer him but to keep him comfortable. That had been her goal throughout this aliment. She could not care for him at home, that's why he was brought to a nursing home. But now here also it became a literal dead end. In the next few days he stopped eating completely.

"Mrs. Joshi, I hope you understand. Madhukar is a diabetic patient, if he stops eating, that will be the end of him." The doctor's declaration pounded not just in her ears but her heart too.

Just a few days ago she gave him the consent to leave this world. Those words turned into venom now. Did he really listen to her? Or was it just a coincidence? Nurse Sue kept assuring her with her usual kind words, "Jyoti it's not your fault, the disease has reached the last step now." This knowledge could not console her.

Just then Emily, the dietician, walked into the room. Emily had always tried to accommodate Madhukar's diet per Jyoti's requests. She was keen on making sure that he would get the food he was used to at home.

"We are aware of our hunger and thirst because our brain sends us a signal. With his condition the brain has stopped giving those commands. So, he does not feel hungry like we do. Trust me, he is not going to be aware of that. He is beyond that now." Jyoti's ears could not absorb Emily's words.

'The taste of food remains until our last breath,' Jyoti remembered lines from *Bhagavad Geeta*. But another social worker had told her, "Hearing continues until the last breath." Who do I believe? The tempest in Jyoti's mind churned.

"Jyoti, you have taken such a good care of him that I wish other family members could follow your example. You are my role model. I am sure he still feels deep down, your love and devotion for him. That is why he is calm and content. Look at how angry the other patients are, constantly screaming. Now his end is coming nearer but let me tell you it will be very calm. Trust me, all the credit goes to you Jyoti," Emily kept talking.

Jyoti moaned to herself. In the beginning when his personality lost its tenderness, his soft voice and loving words all got wiped out and he used to start yelling at her. His harsh voice not only scratched her heart but also the walls of their home.

Her ears ached for his soft whispers. She would even take his shouting full heartedly now. She thirstily longed to hear him speak. Her spirit plummeted into darkness. She had never experienced such deep despair ever before. She knew the reason… 'You are my sun', she used to tell him lovingly, but now her sun is swallowed by the clouds. She remembered Sant Dnyaneshwar's famous lines, '*Janiv neniv bhagwanti* nahi.' The ultimate truth is beyond consciousness. Did Madhukar really reach that stage? Does he really not feel all this pain that I feel for him? She started choking on her tears. Her mind had cracked so many times over his sufferings. She was afraid that one more crack would shatter her mind into millions of shards.

***

She wiped her tears streaming down her cheeks, and as usual made sure that he would not see her cry. A gentle pat on his back, she gave his charge to the nurse and quickly left his room. Started her car mechanically to go home. But before she noticed, the tires steered in a different direction.

Just the other day the social worker Melanie had asked if she had done any provision for his final rights. She had only nodded and avoided discussing it further. But in reality, about a month ago she had determinedly looked online at the local funeral homes that had facilities for cremation. Still she could not gather her courage to go visit them. Her car sped fiercely and came to a full stop right in front of the white building of Helmes Funeral Home. She entered inside in a daze. "I think the time has come for my husband."

The funeral director could hardly hear her murmurs. But somehow, she managed to ask him all the details of cremation. Madhukar and she had decided to donate their organs to the Framingham Heart Study a long time ago. "One more thing, I want to donate his brain for Alzheimer's research. Do you have the facility for this purpose?"

"Yes, we have done that kind of service many times here before," he assured her calmly, explaining the whole process.

With a heavy heart she started driving towards the home. On the way there was an Indian store. "Jyoti do you have Ganga Jal[35]? You can get it in any Indian store," her friend Rekha's words rained on her charred mind.

---

[35] It is a belief of Hindus that by drinking holy Ganga river's water at the time of your death, it purifies you and helps to take you to heaven.

She stopped the car right in front of the store and hurriedly went in. She had never seen Ganga jal bottles in the store before; there was never in a need to look. But today as soon as she entered, like a boon she saw the bottle on the shelf right in front of her. Is it really pure water from the holy Ganga river? She had surrendered to all those superstitions. Usually her logical thinking mind would have all kind of doubts. But while coping with his illness, all those customs pounded into her from childhood started surfacing and giving her unusual strength.

'Ees jalaka aachman ho, jab pran tanase nikale... Shivase man sharan ho jab pran tanase nikale'-let your soul drink this holy water of river Ganga, when you are on your last journey. Your body-mind-soul will be purified to complete Shiva-bliss', *her favorite bhajan resonated.*

She quietly purchased the bottle and escaped from the store. In the evening sky a loud cry echoed with a string of cranes flying towards the south. Soon winter would rule over and deport the Sun to the southern hemisphere. How do these birds know which way is south? Why don't I have their compass? My sun is going to set forever, where would I go to find his warmth?

Evening spread as the sun was setting. Usually she wound be transcended into that scarlet beauty with complete peace. But today those rays ignited forcefully into her mind. Suddenly she pushed on the brakes and pulled her car over to the side. She started crying ferociously. The twilight's orange and vermilion became more violent and started smoldering her. *I should be with you Madhukar, now every moment.* Her mind declared mutiny.

All her courage went down with the sun disappearing. Dark fear grossed her; without my Raja, my life will be just one long unending wasteland. Her charred mind was thirsty for him as the scorched earth waits for the monsoon. Immediately she turned her car back towards Orchards.

The dinner tray went back with its cover closed, untouched. He did not even look at his supper, nor did she insist on feeding him. Around eight o'clock he fell asleep, and defenselessly she went home. She had not eaten the whole day. Suddenly a volcano emerged in her stomach. But that fire was not from hunger. It was the inferno that was swallowing her beloved.

The phone was ringing as she opened her door. Orchards' caller ID was on the screen. Her heart missed a beat. *I just came from there, why are they calling me?* Nurse Dotty assured her that there was nothing to worry. He was having a little difficulty in breathing, so she needed Jyoti's permission to give him supplementary oxygen. She would have given her own *prana* for him. She replied to Dotty impatiently, "Yes of course, by all means." The phone clicked. But she wanted to hold on to that line, the only connection between her and her beloved.

While sleep bellowed, 'no, no, no' to her tired eyes, she reminded herself, 'Madhukar's birthday is tomorrow.'

***

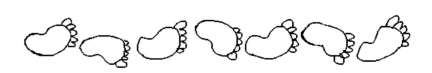

Kojagiri - October 7, 2014

The moon was still struggling to hold on to the night against the light of dawn. The thought that he won't be home to celebrate this Kojagiri, my mind like turned into Amavasya, the no-moon period.

I long for the full bright moon of Kojagiri.
And yearn for the constant blooms of spring.
I crave for a cool breeze to calm the storms.
I need the bird's songs to soothe me.
And the soft tender green grass in the back yard.
Let the wetlands drip onto my mind's scorched desert.
Let there always be sun rising on my horizon.

I crave for my cup to be always full.
Let the hiccups of joy keep coming.
I long to hold my beloved's hand,
Let him be near my side like a constant shadow.

The phone shrilled. *Who is calling so early in the morning?* I pull the blanket over on my head like an ostrich in the sand. *I don't want to talk to anybody!*

"Isn't it his birthday today?" Sumati was on the phone.

"Sumati, he is holding on to his last breath."

"Jyoti today is Kojagiri, a perfect day for him to go."

"Oh, no Sumati no, my Kojagiri will be turning into Amavasya?" I protested and hung up the phone, not even saying goodbye to her.

Eager Abhisarika, pushed away the blanket. Today I decided to wear the diamond studded Mangalsutra, his surprise gift on our first month anniversary of our wedding. I went to the closet. All my beautiful saris were neatly hanging in isolation. I had stopped wearing them for a long time now. No occasion for a pure silk with gold and silver.

"Why don't you wear a sari today?" I heard Madhukar's whispers. He would always ask me when we were going out for an evening. Obediently I started looking for his favorite one. Aha I found it. My hand unfolded that old sari, as did the memories. On one of my visits to Aai, that was the time I was fascinated by yoga philosophy. I was learning the tremendous power of mind. So, I decided to do a little experiment. Romantically, I told Madhukar,

"Raja, Boston to Pune is such thousands of miles apart but we can cross it in a moment. Every dawn when we are awake, and just before we fall asleep at night, there is a zone in which we are neither awake nor asleep. In that luminous state of mind, let's send each other one particular color every day, without uttering a word to each other on the phone! Later in person, we have to guess it."

Once I reached Pune, I started sending the color without a miss through ESP. That time I was still very much in buying beautiful saris, very particular to wear something different than the usual norm. So I went looking for a white sari with an olive-green border. I went all over the shops in Pune and Mumbai only to be disappointed and empty handed. Finally, it was time to return home. Heavy heartedly, one foot still lingering at my ageing Aai's home, I left.

On the return flight, thinking of all the month's unfinished chores, unpaid bills, my job and responsibilities waiting for me in Framingham made me even more anxious. As soon as I entered the house, Madhukar handed me a colorfully wrapped present, "Open it. I saw this and thought of you."

My heart began to dance. He must have missed me too. This darling husband of mine might forget my birthday but he always showered me with presents after our long separation. I eagerly opened the package. Inside was a beautiful white silk sari with an olive-green border! I jumped with joy,

"Oh my god, how did you know I was looking for this combination?"

So, it did work, our mental telepathy was successful. I had been sending him the color of *turmeric*, while I was obsessed with the white sari and olive-green border, and his mind picked up that subconscious signal.

"See, we are always connected no matter how physically far apart we are," I melted in his embrace.

My mind kept chanting only one mantra, *'Raja, When I do Arti*[36] *for you today, just give me one present, the precious jewel of your existence.*

The plate of his favorite homemade *burphi* that I had made, was sitting on the table. Today I was not going to worry about his sugar level. *Burphi* was so soft that it would melt in his mouth, easy to swallow. Its softness reminded me of Madhukar's tender touch, his

---

[36] Aarti is showing a lighted oil lamp before the deities in a spirit of humility and gratitude. Women also do Aarti to their loved ones - father, husband, son, or a brother to honor. Then that person gives them some form of a present to show their appreciation for receiving the special honor.

smiles, and his gentle murmurs. All his colorful memories rolled into a magical flying carpet, taking me for a ride all the way to his nursing home. Today's full moon would be just for two of us. But when I walked in, his room was full of all the people who cared for him; they were all gathered to celebrate his birthday too. I knew it was a protocol in the nursing home. The room was decorated with balloons and flowers. Swati and Chitra entered right after me, taking a little break from their busy day at work.

His frail face he looked even thinner than yesterday. My optimism diminished in his closed eyes. As usual he was not aware of what was happening in the room. His caregiver Loretta, the only one I really always liked, allowed me to light the *Diya*. She popped some pillows behind him to help him sit upright. The motion stirred him to open his eyes like a newborn baby, just for a second. I put the *tilak* on his forehead. Started doing Aarti, he stared at the Diya. I thought, it soothed him and made him happy. But it was only my fantasy. His eyes refused to reflect the sparkle of the little flame. He closed his eyes again, went into a deep sleep.

"Raja, please, I am begging you, give me this day." I whispered in his ears.

The memories of the past removed the cloudy sky and let me ride on the rainbow of our happy life together. A hint of smile on his face, was it my imagination? I rubbed the *burphi* on his withered lips, wondering if he could taste the sweetness?

Loretta helped him back to be comfortable, flat on the bed. She patted my shoulder and left silently; others followed her. The girls kissed their father gently, gave me a tight squeeze. I couldn't help but notice Swati swallowing her own sobs. Chitra hugged me with a forced smile…her lips quivering, "happy birthday *Father-Father.*" She always called him that lovingly after hearing it in P.L. Deshpande's play.

Bidding us goodbye, they both fled the room leaving me all alone. I felt very helpless that I couldn't wipe their sorrow away.

I held Madhukar's limp hand in mine, pretended he was holding my hand too like old days and started reading him from *'The Love Song of J. Alfred Prufrock' by* T.S. Eliot.

He had read it to me the very next day, we were married. I humbly confessed to him that I only understood the gist of it. We continued sharing poetry with each other until he got sick.

Let us go then, you and I when the evening is spread out against the sky.

But I could not continue it. My mind started reciting another poem... Last week I was at the writer's club meeting. Our assignment was *to 'look for the seventh book on the shelf, open the seventh page and read down the seventh line, then make a poem around that sentence.'* What a coincidence! With my luck I got the same T.S. Eliot poem. And then I wrote a vastly different poem...the seventh line by T. S. Eliot was 'to have bitten off the matter with a smile...'

Life has taken a 360 turn on my journey.
We travel together catching the twinkling dreams.
But the laughter, the giggles and love have disappeared
Now in the darkness of nightfall,
All that is left, only the void of your hushed shadow.
If only I did not have the taste of honey,
The poison of your confusion would have been a lot easier to swallow.

I did not notice when his hand slipped away from mine. Destiny unraveled our knot. Now there was only one thing left in my hands, to keep him as comfortable as I can. His breathing grew ragged, I asked the nurse to prop the pillows back up again. I clasped his hand in mine again tightly, hoping to keep him with me forever. His soft touch, still the same as he held my hand, the very first time during *Saptapadi, s*pread moonshine all over my being. Time stood still. The clock forgot to tick. Don't know how long I sat there. Would he be there by my side tomorrow? The night was about to fall. I collapsed into the darkness of unknown. My heart defiantly shrugged away all those callous questions and shouted...

This Kojagiri is ours. This Kojagiri is ours.
The beautiful autumn full moon!
The poetic Sharad-Chandra! Our 47th together,
Bestowing countless blessings
Showing us the beauty on path.
In its mesmeric silver-golden hue.
I will store today forever and live this most beautiful moment with you!
You are here with me exclusively.
Just for me!
No book distracting you, no NPR calling you.
No corporate residues from the day…
and above all, no inanimate mistress called your computer!
How did it happen, my love?
When did I get to claim this space so close to you,
and your undivided attention?
This Kojagiri!
In search of respite from suffering, and the long-gone restfulness,
You are lost in deep sleep.
Far away from me, and the world of mortals.
You show no outward cognizance that I am here,
Holding your hand and your hand is so soft and pale,
And I can hold it for as long as I want
and tenderly reminisce about our saptapadi
when we held hands first time in this life,
and walked seven steps together.
The soft touch of your hand
comes to me as if it were yesterday.
How tightly you held my hand,
not letting me go.
So here I am today,
At your side looking,
holding your soft hand
The exclusive you and your hand
Are my blessings on this Kojagiri
I am trying to be one with you
as we both breathe.
But you are way ahead.
Just can't keep up with you!
What else is new, wasn't that the story always

On all our walks in the woods,
me seven steps behind?
The Seven sacred steps of a Pativrata?
or just the less fit me?
Today, I hold your hand and watch you
'all Mine',
And let memories run through me
sprinkling fulfillment and joy on my parched soul,
Keeping me alive
Ever so undivided, you are my captive!!
Today I am not sharing you with anyone else.
This is my bliss.
My Ultimate bliss
This Kojagiri is indeed only for us.

***

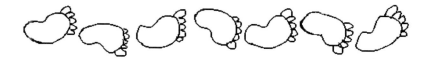

To have and to hold from this day forward, for better, for worse, for richer, for poorer, in sickness and in health, until death do us part. - vows from a Christian wedding

October 9, 2014

10 a.m.

Since he lost his consciousness yesterday, her feet refused to leave him. His nurse Linda started giving him morphine shots. She told Chitra about her decision to stay overnight by his side. But it was vetoed by both girls. "Aai, I know you have to take care of your aching back, so you need a full night's sleep, whereas I can sleep anywhere. I already brought my stuff with me; told my boss that I might be late tomorrow." Swati wouldn't budge and Chitra agreed with her instantly.

But Linda told us, "Now you all listen to me, sometimes the patient does not want to hurt his loved ones. So, they wait until they are not in the room to leave this world. Don't worry, Jyoti I promise you, I will not leave him alone. You all go home and try to get some sleep. If I see him getting worse, I will call. I am begging you."

Helplessly, Jyoti went with Chitra, determined to come back very early in the morning. Swati also returned home reluctantly. This was against all of their wishes. Jyoti stayed that night at Chitra's house. Anxiety cling to her like a thistle. Not a wink, tossing and turning. Earth's axes had shifted and Madhukar's feeble body disappearing from her horizon. Finally, before the crack of dawn, she abandoned her bed and got ready at 6 a.m. Just then the phone penetrated the silence. Trembling, she managed to pick it up. It was Linda, "Come right away." The phone slipped from her hands, without even a reply to Linda, but with the speed of the arrow she ran to Chitra's room. The sleepless night was engraved all over on Chitra's fatigued face. Chitra called Swati immediately. Jyoti knew, even though Chitra told Swati to take a taxi, that Swati would be already on the road driving with the speed of a rocket.

Jyoti insisted on driving, "Chitra you eat your breakfast in the car. Don't know what this day will bring to us! Prepare yourself...we might not even see Daddy alive. You girls have been such wonderful daughters, taking care of him and me too. He knows that. He and I are immensely proud of you."

She decided to take the inside roads instead of highway. The red light blocked her car as usual. Nobody was on the local road at such early morning. She was tempted to go through the traffic light, not to follow the speed limit and soar to his nursing home. But even then, she could not disobey her *samskara*.

The flames of her anguish mixed with the vermilion sky. She got mad at the rising sun. at her inability to stop the universe. Across the highway the traffic was going beyond the speed limits. Somewhere she heard shrilling of a police car. The world was churning as always. Everybody was busy with their own agenda. She wanted to scream at all of them, '*Aren't you ashamed of yourself? My beloved is on the threshold of the death...and you all are carrying on as usual?*'

In that agony somehow, she borrowed the strength to hold on to the steering wheel and turned the knob of the radio. *Kishori's* CD came on, and the melody of morning *raga Bibhas* started plying, it always made her feel calm. The agony in her mind started evaporating with the darkness of the leftover night. Kishori's melodious singing-*saguna* cradled her gently. She was experiencing unusual peace. The warm rays of the rising sun raised another memory. She recognized this state of mind, the same *shakti* she had found ten years ago, that morning when she bid a final goodbye to her Aai.

Out of nowhere her angel, a blue heron landed the nearby pond to give her a *darshan.* In McKinney, Texas, the same symphony of flapping wings, the mark of vermilion around the eye. She realized, lately she had not seen her heron. "I know you will come. Now everything is in your hands…please help my beloved to cross effortlessly," she prayed.

***

Chitra and she both finally reached his ward. Her feeble fingers started tapping the secret code while secretly she wished to crash the door in to save those few seconds. As soon as the door opened, she frightenedly looked at Linda… "*Is he still…?*" Linda nodded.

She forgot to breath for a moment and soared like an arrow to his room. He looked even more frail, like a wilted flower, eyes closed…breathing very slow.

"*Om Tryabakam yajamane sugandhim pushtivardhanam*[37]." Soft chanting was playing in the room.

"Loretta, how did you know the right CD to put on at a time like this?" she wondered, silently patting Loretta's back. Her eyes welled. The last two days his room echoed constantly with all the *stotras*: *Vishnusahastranam, Mrityunjaya mantra, Shiva bhajans, devi sutra.* She believed in all these mantra's power.

"Thank you, thank you so much," she did *namaskar* to Loretta. "Oh, whatever came to my hands, I just put on that CD. Jyoti, I have always seen you putting music on as soon as you enter the room. I also like it and I notice that it helps me to be calm and stay focused," Loretta admitted.

His face so pale it was almost ash gray. Eyes sunken deeply. All the muscles on his face vanished overnight giving way to the skeleton; his face was all prominent bone. She gasped. She felt that her soul was being exchanged for his last breath.

---

[37] Mrityunjaya mantra is the death-conquering mantra, used for contemplation and meditation.

She started stroking his forehead gently, murmuring to him in a very soft tone, "*Raja,* you are not alone. I am right here beside you. I will never let go of your hand." Hanging on the lifeline of his palm she made her grip tighter.

How can I send my beloved to his last journey alone? She always was amused by all the mythological stories of Hindu scriptures but had never really gave them much credence. To her they were simply fables. But at this crucial moment she utterly understood *Sati Savitri's* [38] determination and the magnitude of her devotion to her husband. She wonders whether she could do the same as Savitri and follow Madhukar to the gates of Yama's domain. She was ready to go with him on his further journey. There was not a trace of suicide in her mind.

That very moment Swati entered the room. So quickly? She could not imagine what speed Swati was driving. But she forgot to get angry at her daughter, she could see from Swati's distressed tired face, that she also had a sleepless night like her sister. "Aai, your angel blue heron visited me, saluting with his vast wings as I was coming here," Swati tried to encourage her mother. She thanked the bird again and again for giving her daughter that *shakti*.

Three women who loved him most in the world. Chitra stood on the left side of his bed and Swati sat on his right near his pillow. "Don't be afraid *Raja,* we are with you, you are not alone," she kept repeating in his ears, even though he was beyond hearing. The pendulum kept swinging only forward. Mark arrived within a few minutes. His 6-foot-tall frame like a fortress tower. But there was no more fortress to win. She had lost the war. Still, seeing him by her side gave her some comfort.

Clock on the wall showed the time: 10:10 a.m. His breathing stopped. So it seemed, did time.

Awghachi rang ek zala.
Rangi rangala shreerang

---

[38] Savitri was a princess, who married an exiled prince named Satyawan, who prophesied to die early. The legend describes Savitri's wit and love, which saved her husband from the death god Yama

All the colors became one.
Merged into Krishna 'consciousness'

So ham asmi[39],
So ham asmi.

I am that Supreme Brahman-the energy,
I am that Supreme Brahman-the energy.

Her eyes saw when the prana left his body. She also felt when the urja, energy, in him fled. The peace in her mind stayed put. Birth and death are two sides of the same coin. The same inexplicable peace as when she witnessed her mother's last moment.

***

He died very peacefully, without any complications. His darling daughters, favorite son-in-law and I were all standing right next to him until his last breath. For a long time nobody uttered a word or moved. But I can't feel that peace anymore. Mourning spreads like a tidal flood. *'You were supposed to go with him! You are no Savitri!'* My wounded mind accused, ashamed of my failure.

"Ambe Jagdambe, please release him from his suffering." This was my constant appeal for the last few months. Now I can't bear the Goddess's answers to my prayers. The bitter poisonous taste, my mouth went dry. I forced myself to open my eyes. The room is exactly the same. Nothing has changed. Same old furniture, curtains, lamp, everything in the same place. His lifeless body also is still here. Then why does my life feel like a wheel disconnected from a vehicle, tumbling on a slope in the opposite direction? The brakes are not working, and I have lost control. My beautiful *sansar* has collapsed in seconds like a palace built from a deck of cards. Now sorrow clings to me like a leech. What would I

---

[39] In Vedic philosophy it means identifying oneself with the universe or ultimate reality.

do? How would I survive all alone? How can I start a new life without my beloved? The bereavement pierced me like hundreds of a bee sting.

Many years back, I was watering the garden in our Framingham backyard. I did not see the bees' nest in the ground, and by mistake I stepped on it. The cloud of bees rose wildly and started stinging me from all directions. I painfully danced the *Tandav nrutya* for the next 24 hours. How many hours- days- months- years would it take to get over Madhukar's departure? My body and mind were on fire. I felt a choking sensation. My hand went to my throat, suddenly my fingers grasped the *Mangal sutra* beads around my neck. He had put that on me in front of all the wedding guests and *Agni* as witnesses. I took it off and put it into his inert hand, forced his fist to be closed over it, never to let it out. I released him from my bondage.

'*Dharmech arthech naati charami*' [40]

I gathered my courage to move away from him. I noticed a vague presence of somebody behind me. I turned around to see a line of people standing against the wall paying homage to my brave fallen warrior. Another protocol of the nursing home. Still all these caregivers became his new family at the Orchards nursing home. After all, they did take care of him. As the months passed, I learned to appreciate their help. I bowed to them, thanking them, overwhelmed with gratitude. They all left quietly one by one to resume their duty to care for others.

I turned the CD player on. I wanted the room to fill with *Shanti Mantra* for his last voyage and good vibes for the next occupant of this room. The door closed as the girls quietly left me alone for few minutes with him, taking all the light away. His passing liberated him from that dreadful disease but same time it locked me into a solitary confinement.

Soon the van from funeral home had arrived. Two men moved his body into a coffin on wheels and started pushing it towards the main

---

[40] Under any circumstances, I shall not depart or separate in life from you, and I will follow the path of Dharma, the righteous way - the bridegroom vows to his bride at the seven steps of saptapadi.

door. We all rushed to help them, but Loretta stopped me gently. "Jyoti, remember, I welcomed him on his very first day, it is my job to escort him to the van on his last day also." Feebly we followed while my mind wailed in silence.

Finally, in the end one of us is gone,
You have gone much further ahead.
Just a point on a horizon,
and I am seven lives behind you.
Tears are dried. Mind is void.
The memories are blocking my way.
The vast distant of eternity
I must find a time travel machine.

As promised, Loretta carefully helped to put his coffin in the van. In a strangely aloof state of mind the four of us returned to his empty room. Chitra and Swati had carefully decorated their father's room so he would be surrounded by familiar things from our home: family photos, my paintings, his favorite books, etc. The ambiance of the room felt like an altar with the religious idols missing. My darling daughters hurriedly gathered all his belongings and tucked them away in the suitcase. I signaled the girls to leave the room so I can be alone. Don't know how long I just sat on the chair, feeling numb. Overcast sky, rain afraid to fall, as my footsteps reluctantly to leave his room.

Some bizarre *shakti* empowered me. I ran out of the room. So many people had helped him: the cleaning lady, the laundryman, the cook, the nurses, social worker Melanie.

"You took such good care of my husband. I am in your debt forever, thank you, thank you," I kept repeating to them on my way out. I told Chitra to order pizza for the day and nighttime caregivers for the next two days. I reached the main gate in a daze. I did not want to stay in that building even for a second longer.

I pushed the door open to face the remainder of my life. Just then the receptionist came running to me. Her kind words almost made me stumble, "Jyoti, wait! I will always remember your singing to Dr. J. Not only it calmed him down, but it helped other residents also and most of all, it tremendously helped me too."

I could not help but laugh. Me, singing? Then I remembered. When I used to take Madhukar in his wheelchair for a walk every day, I would whisper the prayer chants. I had no idea that anybody else heard me.

The caravan of our individual cars started going towards the Funeral home. The thought of his body locked up in the coffin all alone, made me shiver and feel suffocated. Chitra stopped at the town hall to register her father's death. Without a death certificate we wouldn't be able to get his body back for cremation.

***

Finally, we reached home. For a long ten months the house was not used to Madhukar anymore, yet still today it felt even emptier. The walls began to close in on me, like a prison. I begged my daughters, "Please take me to Borderland Park," as if I expected to find him there. On our way there, we picked up Jeevan early from school.

I sat on our favorite rock by the lake. The leaves were painted in autumn colors. The landscape consoled me. My mind began to calm down. But it only lasted for a few moments like the ripples on the water. Even though my brain knew the reality, my heart was not ready to accept the truth yet.

We returned in the afternoon. I told Chitra to go home. Told Swati the same, her cat Keshoba must be waiting for her. But she refused. She looks strong but I know it's only a facade. Secretly I was happy to have her by my side, I did not want to be alone that day. That night we both sank into a deep exhausted sleep, I wonder like a snake shades his skin, if all the stress of the last five, six, seven years had dropped away.

***

Madhukar will always be buried deep in my heart. Still, the feeling that he is no more on this earth tortured me. Tears continuously streamed. I moved around lifelessly for entire days, eyes continuously streaming. For the last nine months I was not living with him so I should be used to the empty house by now. Why am I so saddened by his absence? All my life I had studied the philosophy of *Vedanta*, but now when I needed it most, all the wisdom evaporated. What happened to *shanti* that I found when the prana left his body? Then that *shanti* was so ingrained in me, but now it only remains like a shadow under my foot.

***

With a gloomy mind I started moving like a robot, doing my everyday chores as if they were a punishment. Swimming, going for walks and yoga practice continued without usual interest. Whenever I would sit for meditation then tears would flow fiercely as if a dam burst opened. So I stopped doing it. I was a living ghost.

One evening I returned from my walk; it was a struggle to enter the dark house. I ran crazily turning on every single light- the table lamp, ceiling light, bed side, on the top of the stove, in the bathroom…not a single light was left off in the rooms. Still my eyes could not see any light. I could not find solace. I reached for the CD player…my favorite bandish- song- was on it already, '*My beloved has gone out of the country leaving me all alone. Oh beloved give me your darshan! The day and nights are long. I can't live a single moment without him anymore. Oh beloved please come back to me!*'

My hands froze to turn it on. All the classical music became like venom of a snake bite; the melody that once used to caress me has become the sharp thorns giving a blood bath. Only the mehfil of sadness remained.

Blanket, TV, remote, books, to the hammer nails become alive with Madhukar's touch… now floundering to me. House full of things but it felt empty and bleak. Memories stormed in everything- everywhere. I could not face them. "Why are you punishing me?" I kept asking him again and again, as usual he kept silent.

The phone rang constantly, "*Our deepest condolences… sorry for your loss.*" The doorbell announced the arrival of friends with the same words, "*I am so sorry… How are you coping alone?*" I knew that all the callers meant well. But then the tender scab from the wound would open and begin to bleed.

***

His body was still in the coffin at the funeral home waiting to be cremated. The lifeless body had to follow the rules. According to Massachusetts law, one can't do the final rites until the death certificate is in your hands. Even though his demise was registered on the very same day, it followed by a weekend. It hadn't yet been five days since he died.

It was 4:00 a.m. I was still awake. This was not new to me. My sleep had parched since he became ill. The dawn muddled with darkness from my mind, still blind, my eyes could not see the sunrays.

The laughter that went through the entire octave has taken a vow of silence.
No more snoring that croons in musical notes, game of intellect is over.
Mischievous sneezing that tremors the earth, blended in muteness.
No more rat race, pointless pursuits. No more schedules.
Empty walls are missing the loving stares.
No more office projects, pursuits. No more schedules.
The humble wisdom of awareness, the contest for prizes, crazy mind has calmed down.
No mountains to climb, no confinement to the wheelchair.
No more 4 wheels 2 wheels or ankle express. No speed limits.
The detention by the nursing home's locks has been knocked down.
No more science fiction. The reality begins.
Creator has taken the appreciator. Awareness is wiped out.
The curtain came down on the ballet of hammer and nails; the cruel thrashing by the horrible disease has ended.
The gardener abandoned his blossoming garden. No more wasteland in a barren mind.
Gastronomical paradise has dried up and so has the bitter medicine. Indulgence of ice cream or juggling of sugar measurements. No more... no more.
Where is the loving dad? Grandson is waiting impatiently.
Finally the fat lady wailed, drenching loneliness has dried up.

The companion has quit the journey, overflowing love tipped over into salty ocean of
Tears.
Now only defeated words remain, and finally, silenced breaths.

***

Rahana nahi des virana hai - I don't want to live here, this land is foreign. - Kabir

October 13, 2014, my birthday

It has been a week since Madhukar passed away. "Please promise me that you won't give me the cruel gift of your exodus on my birthday. I will never forgive you," I was begging him while he was on his death bed. He must have heard me and quietly left before my birthday. Tomorrow we will do his last rites. I will have to say my final goodbye to him. That thought is agonizing. Madhukar used to officiate weddings, thread ceremony, Satyanarayana, wastushanti, all of the rituals for the Hindu community. Still we both knew that we did not want any antya samskara, the rituals of death in the end. Every time I asked him about it, he would skillfully avoid the subject. So I really had no idea what to do tomorrow.

October 14, 2014

"Swatu, go for a long walk, then your stress will go away. Keep your daily routine. You will feel better. This is not just my experience, but it is proven by scientific research. The adrenaline that is created by physical exercise helps to release stress and the brain gets rejuvenated," I was talking to Swati on the phone.

I remember after hearing the news of my dear Dada's demise, I went to work right away. I needed to follow my daily rituals. So today I decided to go for a swim. Any kind of speed churns my mind into creativity -out of that sometimes a painting, poem or an idea for a project is born.

This was always my reward. The same thing happened today while my body was making waves in the pool.

On the way to Holiday Inn, the rhythmic speed of the car put my mind into creative gear. I became alive with *shakti* to know, how I would conduct Madhukar's last rites later that morning. I was able to focus. I scribbled everything down on the piece of paper as soon as I came home. I decided to wear the white sari that Rekha had given me.

***

"Raja, you chose the right muhurta for your final journey," my mind murmured as Chitra parked the car at the crematory. We first moved to Boston in the same month of October. Our most favorite season. Glowing sunrays whispering into autumn mornings. Fall colors bursting through the leaves, singing a finale.

There were lots of cars already crowded in the parking lot. I am a follower of Dr. Leo Buscaglia, so I always hug people when I see them. But when I saw my friends' hands reaching for me to give a hug, I begged the girls to tell them that their loving touch would make me cry. I desperately wanted to have a few moments alone.

As Keats would have said, "*the Vale of Soul-Making.*" My raja and I, we started walking side by side together again. We had begun this beautiful journey of seven steps long time ago, turning into millions of steps. Today it's our final *saptpadi*.

The red maple was signaling to me from the corner ahead, the colorful carpet of falling leaves. I bent down to collect some pretty leaves from nature's rangoli and went inside the crematory to his coffin. Remembering all the promises from saptapadi, I started putting each leaf on his coffin. Exactly at the seventh vow, no more leaves remained in my hands. Was this a coincidence?

"Madhukar, I entered in your life smilingly, my hand in your hand…today with the same smile, I am giving you my final *nirop*-wishing you smooth sailing. So please don't worry about me or our daughters. You had given me so much in life up to the rim…that will last me for the next seven lives."

I could not make out who was reciting the words of Shankaracharya's that came out of me,

'*Name mrutyushanka neme jatibhedah: pita naiv me naiv mata na janmaH:*
Chidanandrupah Shivoham Shivoham.

I have no fear of death, nor have I any distinction of Caste.
I have neither father nor a mother-nor even birth
I am pure knowledge & bliss, I am all auspiciousness, I am Shiva the pure.'

I signaled the girls and Mark. Jeevan joined them instantly. All of them pushed his wooden coffin gently towards the electric fire. Jeevan stood on his toes to reach the button on the door. The fire diminished Madhukarjyoti's saga of companionship in a split second. With a heavy heart I stumbled in the corner of the room, not knowing what to do or where to go. One by one from the line, people started moving towards me. My numbed mind could not make out or feel their compassionate words, but their loving hugs opened the doors of my controlled willpower and the torrent of tears started flowing profoundly.

We all returned back to our home in Norton. Swati had arranged all pictures of her father around the house. The camera was best at showing off his hearty laughter, gusto on his handsome face…meekly trying to bring him back to life. I got trapped in the labyrinth of those photos, forgetting the cruel reality. Swirling laughter in the room brought me back to the bitter truth. Everybody was seeing Madhukar's past with a new touch. Remembering his funny jokes and absent-mindedness. The walls so desperately needed to hear that sound of joy; they were silenced without it for a long nine months. I did not notice when my friends Meena, Pushpa, and Suniti took over the meals to feed the guests. I would be in their debt forever.

Suddenly fatigue overpowered me. I kept babbling continuously, talking to friends as if nothing had happened. Many years ago I was doing the same thing - after I was awake from the gas that dentist gave me for tooth extraction. The brain is weird. Same thing happened after my baby Swati was born; I started chattering without stopping. My body exhausted after giving birth, but still happy. That new life filled my universe with ecstasy. I felt bigger than the sky! But today… one life had vanished leaving a huge vacuum in my life with a vast chasm. And still I kept jabbering.

The sun rises every day while dissolving my days, my spirit plummeting into the dusk always. I made up my mind and decided to throw away this heavy blanket of darkness from my mind.

"Let's pay our respect to Daddy by giving him a warm memorial. Let's celebrate his life."

I firmly told the girls and they could not agree with me more. I started looking for a suitable hall. Lots of our friends would have to travel from far, so there should be some delicious refreshments. '*Whatever you do, do it the best you can, and full heartedly*', remembering my Aai's coaching I threw myself in the process. I found a way to keep my impaired mind busy. I planned the entire program from choosing a caterer to composing the program sheet for that day. I started gaining my confidence back slowly, still sometimes finding myself in a rut.

***

"I feel like a bumblebee who does not know that he cannot fly. This helps me to do things that I never knew that I couldn't!" - Madhukar Joshi

November 9, 2014

The church hall was packed with our friends. Seeing them in such a large number, I was overwhelmed and a little timid. I tried my best to not to shed tears. Mark welcomed all the people with a short introduction about the program.

"Now I'm going to play Ajoba's favorite symphony, Beethoven's 'Ode to Joy,'" proclaimed ten-year-old Jeevan standing boldly in front all the audience. What an honor to Ajoba. I was so proud of that little munchkin. His fingers caressing softly on the piano keys, a pin drop silence in the hall, followed by Meera Bai's bhajan, *my* favorite. Shuchita's melodious voice filled the hall.

'*Jo tum todo piya mai naahi todu re tori preet tori Krishna, kaun sang jodu?*

My beloved! You have broken the bonds of our love and gone away. But I would never allow my love for you to be shattered. Now where would I look for that precious love! I could never love anybody but you only!

"Thank you Suchita Didi, that was beautiful." Chitra took a deep breath, holding the mike. "Thank you all for joining us here today to honor my father, Madhukar Joshi. It truly means a lot to us, some of you came from so far away. Now I will read you a short poem by Linda Ellis, called 'The Dash'…

1938 – 2014
How do you describe brilliance and success of full 76 years in a dash?
With his sheer intelligence and dedicated hard work, he lived his life with great enthusiasm; you could never say the word "can't" to my dad.
He always said, "When you get lemons you make lemonade!
My dad was a self-made man still he would say very casually about his success,
"I just happened to be in the right place at the right time" …

Chitra kept talking, taking a pause to control her grief. I had to control myself not to run towards her for rescue.

Swati came on the stage next. "Daddy, one day as you were walking in the mall with Ai, you told her, "*I have finally discovered Victoria's gupith (secret).*" When people groan at my puns and Marathi wordplay, they often tell me that I am Madhukar's daughter!" She helped ease the solemn mood by telling funny stories about Madhukar. Hilarious laughter took over the audience. Dear Daddy, we are all gathered here today to celebrate your indomitable spirit. We miss you very much but are glad you are free and at peace…

My mind is like a beehive bursting with your memories.
Your absence stings, but at the same time the joy of our life together gives me a taste of honey over and over again.
You and Ai taught us to be fearless and independent.

You never once told me or Chit that we couldn't do something just because we were girls, but showed us, we could achieve anything we set our minds to.
Daddy, you were a wonderful father and role model for us.
You lived with integrity and stood up for your principles.
For example, you refused to work in a cigarette company even though they had given you a great job offer!
You showed us what "family values" really means,
supporting not just your parents and younger brother back in India but to your daughters and loving us unconditionally no matter what.
You were proud of your roots, and also appreciated this land that welcomed you with so many opportunities.
Your heroes were from both cultures: Shivaji, Dr. Anandibai Joshi, Ramanujan, Lincoln, Mark Twain, Jane Goodall...
You were very prejudiced. (Let me explain what I mean by reading a page from his journal):
> *I am prejudiced against organized religions, orthodox rules, and blind faith!*
> *I am prejudiced against military spending that goes on in a mindless fashion.*
> *I am prejudiced against rulers who try to dictate morality without understanding basic human nature......*

Daddy, you lost your memories, but you will live on in ours.
You stopped being verbal, but your actions continue to speak through us.
You were no longer mobile, but we are walking in your footprints.
You were short in physical stature, but we all looked up to you.
You loved solving math puzzles, but your legacies cannot be counted.
You were born into poverty but left us with riches beyond measure.
Daddy, you loved astronomy, and now you are among the stars.

Our friends Anand and Pushpa started reading some excerpts from the hundreds of condolence letters and memories of Madhukar that the Joshi family was showered with.
I don't know how long they were reading; I was just so numb until I heard Shuchita's soothing melody. She sang Madhukar's favorite bhairavi bhajan, 'Jo *bhaji Hari Ko Sada.*' Shuchita's voice gave me strength. I realized that every single one in the audience had helped me in Madhukar's illness in some ways. This was the time to

acknowledge that. I decided to go on the stage and started addressing everyone gathered.

"It takes a village to nurse a sick person. You all became that village for us. You became our family. I will be always thankful to you all. You have touched our lives in unique ways!" I took out the crumpled note that I had scratched yesterday and started reading it.

Dear Madhukar, this is for you, a final farewell. My memories!

The dawn breaks with the vermilion colors of your memories.
I am walking along the pond, holding your hand like always.
There, my mind hums like a bee trapped inside the beautiful thousand-petal lotus
of your memory.
Raindrops are dancing a garba with the wipers as I start the car on my return.
Your laughter flashes like lightning in my darkened mind.
Your memory illuminates the romantic candle at my lonely dinner table.
Beloved, when I first met you, I was free and liberated.
But now that I have lost you, your love has captivated me.
There is only one reason behind these shackles.
In my lonely Mehfil-recital, behind the melody,
Memories of you are echoing constantly like the Tanpura[41]

***

---

[41] In Indian classical music, a musical drone by the Tanpura is considered to be an essential accompaniment for the musician to stay in tune.

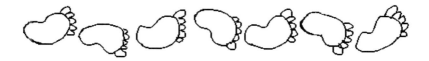

Life begins when the comfort zone disappears. – Unknown

November 10, 2014

I was filling out a form at the bank, and my pen struggled at the very first column. *Please select one: __ married __ widowed __ single.*

A bitter truth in permanent ink, scorning me! "I will not give you an inch of my kingdom," Rani Laxumbai of Jhansi rebounded in my ears. Madhukar whispered softly in my ears, "you are not a frail, incompetent woman." Ahilyabai Holakar, Ramabai Ranade, Laxumbai Tilak, Rashtra Sevika Samiti leader Maushi Kelkar, Indira Sant; one after another they crowded in my mind. I humbly bowed to them and tick marked the 'single' column.

***

I wondered why my oatmeal tasted a little salty this morning. Only to realize my own tears were dripping into the bowl...like the kitchen faucet dripping all night. It would have been fixed instantly, only if you were still around. I opened the curtain to distract myself. It was raining softly, raindrops tapping on the roof top silently, like my own tears. I wondered if the earth was crying to give me company.

The urn of Madhukar's ashes that was just delivered by the funeral home was sitting on the table. Again my tears started flowing. Raja, we were going to travel all around the world. Well then, from now on I am going to sprinkle your ashes in the earth wherever I go. So you will be with me. I left the urn on the table and went for a walk in the neighborhood.

I saw Pam coming across. I quickly wiped my tears and forced a smile. Pam patted on my shoulder and said, "Jyoti, you must be lost without him."

I assure her, "No, I am not lost! No, I am not lost."
Yes! I can find my way through the labyrinth highways to come back to my empty home!
Yes, I can track all the sweets that he was forbidden to taste through the aisles of grocery store to satisfy my craving for sweets.
Of course I am not lost when I change the battery of the smoke alarm that shrills through the stillness of the night.
The mask of composure torn.
But honestly, I am lost. I am lost forever.
When I wake up hysterically crying…Noticing his absence in my bed, only to find his smile trapped in the cold photo frame on my bedside table.
Even though the sky is glittering, I am totally lost without my real Sun.
His diminished existence has cracked my overflowing cup of life.
His constant support has silenced my creativity.
The little constellation is lingering with the moon sliver, making me lost without my mate!
Yes, as I observe the North star, I am totally lost without his guidance,
On my life's compass.

***

January 19, 2015

My darling daughters insisted I travel again. So I went with a group of friends to South Africa. We are on Table Mountain in Cape Town, South Africa. I hurriedly walked towards the plateau before they reached it. A nice niche near the cliff lured me into a meditation spot. I settled down under the blue sky. Mind merging in the surroundings for a few minutes. A gentle breeze of footsteps declared your arrival. How did you know I was here? You were sitting right next to me, cheek to jowl! I felt your bodiless presence covering me. Dissolving in that totality, I sat in silence. The power of divine's infinite contentment spread within me. There was no I - me or mine... you and I are the same. It was a blissful experience.

The hubbub of the tourist brought me back to reality. Suddenly I remember my effort to rush to this spot before everybody. I took out the crumpled plastic bag from my pocket and sprinkled a few of your ashes in the earth. You were resting like a rangoli on the Table Mountain. Remember, I made a promise to you, I will take you with me wherever I go in the world.

"I am here-there. In the shining dew drops, in the torrential of dark clouds. In the valleys and crevasse of the mountain... I am everywhere," Rumi echoes on the cliff.

I returned to hotel, while leaving you resting on the mountain. The room felt empty without you. I stood in the gallery feeling your absence in the surroundings.

Deep green sea, dancing waves. One lost cloud in the blue sky, like my mind wandering aimlessly. I see a sailboat with a gust full of your memories. Far away on the horizon,
nebulous hills next to each other's shoulders, like you were next to me on the Table Mountain. I thought I was going to be all alone. What a fool I was! Did I not know from now on you are my guide?

***

Calendar spinning heartlessly, not caring for the three long months since you left me. While I was traveling, I was at my best. But in this empty house, the hush walls start choking me. I can't bear it. I wander room to room looking for you. Life is playing a game of malice with me. Can't find the purpose of living? I search in the pantry or something in the freezer, stale old food tastelessly chewing, for I don't feel like cooking.

Like moon blossoms, the bud you used to be blossomed the art of living for me. Your intimacy used to flourish my being.

When the cardinal sings on the tree, swinging the branch gently, reminds me once, you used to swing my spirit gently...tears welled up. Your love is sucking all the life force from me.

Blades of grass sprouting from hard frozen earth, tears start shooting from my dormant heart. I choke with a sadness...what's wrong with me?

Only one number is minus from the population of the world...then why the sum of my life remains at zero? Is this the rule of your statistic?

The joy of living is at the speed of a turtle. The memories one by one pour like grains from a silo, suffocating me.

When I turn off the lamp at night, the pillow is soaked in my tears. Sleep washed away in that flood. Dawn rises with showers of tears. How can be so many tears locked in my two eyes?

Tears competing with the notes of a melody, angrily I turned off the CD player. I try to sit quietly but the tears bury my Dhyana. Car wheels turn into our house. Only two grocery bags. For whom? The tears hungrily fill my dinner plate. The empty chair across me, thirsty tears drink all my appetite. I keep drowning in my own tears. I force myself to go to a social gathering. At the thought of entering the hall alone, my foot forbids me to leave the car. I start looking only for one person in that crowd, but I can't find you anywhere!

***

Far away on the horizon, a bonfire of rays started. The birds' loud trumpets woke me up. I jumped from the bed; the clock was showing it was already half past eight. How can I sleep so late? All the morning rituals - or Raja you might call it idiosyncrasies- would have to be skipped. I would be carrying that guilt throughout the day. 'So you woke up late! So what? The world is not going to fall apart!' Your tender tone resonated in my ears. 'Be a free spirit and live the way you used to,' again you urge me. Somewhere along your illness I became very rigid. I needed to keep my day in order to get everything done in time. Do you remember, once we were at the library for a workshop? The speaker gave us only five minutes to make the list of things that we would like to do in life, our hobbies, and passions, etc. *My pen could not keep up with list of my hobbies. Then she asked, so now tell me how many do you do every day? I was embarrassed to tell her that I do them all. Why can't I do the same now?*

Yesterday I saw a man sitting in the car in front of as I was driving. Oh my god, I had to pinch myself because it was you. The same way you use to sit in the car, same hair, same shoulders. "Hey, where are you going without me?" I shouted, my mind racing when I pushed on the gas pedal to get ahead of that car. When I overtook the car, I realized it was only an illusion.

'Giridhar aow na ek bar hamare ghar'...Giridhar please come to my abode one more time!

Jasaraj's singing on the car CD was in its glory. *Give me your darshan. Raja, really please visit me just once.* My crazy mind did not know that just one lick of honey continues the greed, wanting more. When you were alive near my side, I could easily be aloof from you. Now that you are gone, I am engulfed in you like an undertow current. I am mad with anger. Frustrated by my own defeat. I gathered my courage and decided that I am going to learn something new every day. I assembled my shattered life and started living again. Rejoined the writers' group. Attended Zumba class every day at the senior center to rekindle my passion for dancing. Went to book club at the library. Visited art galleries and entered my paintings in exhibitions. Joined Mahjong with the ladies at the club house. One thing I never stopped was swimming. Terry and I started our evening walks. Volunteered in the community. I got involved in life again.

Still, the shadows of dusk would make my heart sad. I would get very restless. Harsh reality would start, and I could not sleep alone in the house. I started watching movies into late at night. All these worldly tools for living were still not enough to fill the void in my life. This was a farce to keep me busy. It would not fill the absence of you, my beloved. You made a huge hole in my life, which I am trying to fill with these mundane things. I am trying so hard but failing every minute. Like a road sign, *'Work in progress, road closed.'* All the roads of my life are closed to repair my broken mind.

***

August 31, 2015

Now Swati and I are on the train to the Canadian Rockies, the trip you and I planned but never went. The train has picked up a slow rhythm. Soft white snow icing sprinkled on the peak tops. Mountains' cliffs stumbling into each other, still, holding hands so tight. Where are they going in such a unity? Native river lost in her reverie. I have a feeling she is going to take a wrong turn. Suddenly a royal eagle soars into the deep indigo sky, lugging my spirit on his wings. Alpine trees stretching their long neck taking your evergreen memories up so high. Joy of all this wonderland is cradled on the leaves of aspen branches. Still I can't find you anywhere. Wounded heart, I search for you hopelessly in the wilderness of valleys and caves. All these beautiful endless range of mountains prevail still just to welcome us. Where are you? You should have been by my side! How in the world you choose this enchanting moment to disappear beyond the horizon without a trace?

Walking along Lake Louise in the Canadian Rockies, I am mesmerized once more by its turquoise water. Melting me in Beirut's sea, the one we saw it together many years ago. Sun rays shimmering on the water making me calm. I kept walking for hours, forgetting my back pain. The sun's setting on the horizon. The shadow turning long under my feet. The lake ends near the base of the mountain. I am sure Swati must have reached a long time ago. I sat on the rock at the edge, quietly took out the little plastic bag and sprinkled your ashes near the gleaming water. I know you would love this place to rest for eternity. The cranes wailing, separated by the lotus leaf from her mate. *'Don't cry when I die. Is he gone? He is no more. Don't grieve in vain!'* Rumi crooning in my ears.

"Aai what are you doing, bending so deep? You will fall into the water," Swati's gentle touch brought me back to my senses.

***

October 7, 2015

I am awake by early morning. As usual I lit the lamp in front of your smiling photo in the altar. Yours was the most handsome picture among the idols and statues of Gods. "*Suprabhatam, Raja! Happy birthday!*" I shouted with joy, as if you were just in the next room. I opened the back door eagerly. Saffron sunrays crinkle on my face, sweetening my soul. His birthday! I am more excited than he would have been. I knew what to cook for Naivedya. His favorite sheera. I became aware that his birthday will follow ruthlessly by Oct 9th, the date I want to rip off from the calendar.

Anna Kendrick's song was playing at Zumba. '*You're gonna to miss me when I'm gone. You're gonna miss me by my hair… when I'm gone!*'

The hide and seek of sun and rain started again by that song. My crazy wounded mind is not cured by any remedy. I began to drown in a bottomless pit. All the philosophy vaporizes away like a camphor. The love fever takes over. Your absence turns into dried wood adding to the inferno of my mind. The world is deaf to my wailing.

I come home. Hang my sweater in the closet that is full all-weather fancy garments. But my favorites are the two London Fog jackets, his and hers, that I bought for his 60th birthday. He always wanted that.
Our 7th home, at last all settled for retreat. Finally a master bedroom bath that has two sinks. I always wanted that. Two electric toothbrushes. His and hers. He always wanted that.
The bedroom now has two walk-in closets, his and hers. I always wanted that.
Above the closet rim adorns a wood carving, 'Mom and Dad'-Chitra made that for an art project in 6th grade. Now our grandson Jeevan would soon be in 6th grade.
My mind dry as a bone, competes with that hard wood. Ready to carve his memories on.
I go to his closet and toss all his clothes in the empty box for Salvation Army.

Who is going to salvage me? I wonder? I never wanted that. I never wanted that.
Months have gone by. His toothbrush vanishes, his sink is parched. My closet is full of untouched fancy clothes.
His closet is vacant like my mind. I never wanted that. I never wanted that.
A long year has gone by.
On one fine sunny day full of your sparkly memories, by mistake I open his closet.
All the empty hangers are dangling.
I snatched a few left-over metal hangers which he always hated.
Bend and twist them in anguish.
About to throw them in the trash.
A figure emerges out of the crooked shapes and tangles.
A nymph sitting on knees, palms folded to her bosom.
Perhaps an angel. Perhaps a Phoenix. Perhaps my muse?
I glide to the backyard. Hang the angel on a Japanese red maple!
The tree was his most favorite. He always wanted that. He always wanted that.
Gentle breeze swings the mental hanger's creation clinking in the trees...
so do his golden memories. Hanging in my mind clinking like wind chimes.
I would want that. Definitely I would want that!

***

October 9, 2015, Raja, your first *punytithi*

Beautiful surroundings of serene nature. Henry David Thoreau's sacred Walden Pond. After many years I am here with Chitra and Jeevan, at Walden Pond, our favorite place. Nature's Bhairavi will start soon. I see colored leaves ready to drop. Fall is in the air. I scattered your Raksha in the woods near the water, my palms sending a prayer into the universe.

'Sarwathra sookhina santhoo, sarwa santhoo niramaya', may all become happy. May all see auspiciousness everywhere.

Your immortal memories bundled up under my arm, I started walking slowly around the pond. Jeevan caught up with me shortly. He taught me how to skip stones on the water. I had a great teacher, so I learned the skill right away.

Swati came in the evening after work, holding long-stem red roses in her hand. "Today our absent-minded (professor) Daddy commanded me to bring these for you." I melted into her hugs. Mark, Chitra and Jeevan reminded us that Daddy's favorite feast at the table is getting cold. This harsh day melted in the celebration of your puns and jokes.

December 27, 2015

Days go by without a trace of you.
Are you still here?
I see a red cardinal sitting still on a dormant tree.
They say cardinals bring memories of loved ones.
So where are those memories?
Are they buried in the frozen winter ground?
Are you still here?
When I light the candle on the dinner table,
The food tastes normal.
My first bites always used to be salty, flavored with my tears.
Are you still here?
At night, eyes heavy with reading, I turn off the light near my bed side.
Sleep comes naturally, taking me into a dreamland.
Oh, I see you smiling at me at last.
I am glad you are still here.

***

Country roads take me home, to the place I belong, West Virginia, mountain mama, take me home, country roads. - John Denver

February 7, 2016

Rays of rising sun started sweeping away the debris of the lingering night's darkness. I was standing in the balcony of my brother's home in Sion in India. The neighborhood was still dreaming silently. I was tempted to go for a walk before the heat starts steaming. It has been two months since I arrived in the land of my birth. The first time I have traveled alone to Mumbai since he passed away. The faraway nest was pulling at me. "My Bharat, my motherland!" don't you always tout proudly to your friends in America? The mind's inquisition began. "Yes, that's true, but I long to return to my home, my enchanted backyard in Norton," I confess meekly. When I returned after my annual visits to Aai, Madhukar would be standing there, his arms wide to welcome me back. Rudely, the truth reminds me - just a few days ago I had strewn his ashes in the river Narmada. So, he won't be in Norton upon my return, with his unconquerable smile. But I knew in my heart...

I know My beloved would be waiting there invisibly
to rejoice spring with me.
My favorite birches would look a little whiter.
Daffodils would be craning their neck a little higher to look for me.
Cardinals would race to the branch before other birds arrive
to sing Raja's love song.
The road is uphill, but I feel unusual strength in my tired feet.
I must return to my home, my own sweet home.

Fasten your seat belts. The red sign was lit in the cabin. I could see from my window the vast Arabian Sea churning. I ruminated on all my walks on the beach at Dadar. The soft sand rubbed like Aai's caresses again on my back. The full moon enticing the mad waves, pulled my youth back. I did not know when the moonlight streaked white on my locks, when the wrinkles from the low tide shore appeared on my face. This pearl of joy in the shell that I found, I must carry it with me carefully from now on.

***

Awakening will find me/through the daily mundane/faith's step in front of tiny step. - Alyssa Underwood

Epilogue

"Today is Monday, Nov 13th, 2017," the radio announced. She turned off the alarm, still sleepy but lingering on the date…It sounded familiar, but why? All of a sudden, those years fluttered by like a deck of cards.

November 13th, 1967, a bleak wintery day in Decatur, Ill. After their 10-day honeymoon in Europe, wandering around free as birds, they had just landed in 'Amrika', the land of golden opportunities. Their taxi brought them through the maze of spotless roads, manicured lawns and houses. Hardly anybody on the streets, quite a contrast to Bombay's streets full of hawkers and pedestrians.

The stale air from the locked windows in the hotel room suffocated her with the reality that she would not see Dada and Aai again for a long time. She burst into tears as she pleaded to her husband, "I do not want to stay here. I don't like this country." He understood, smiled gently and assured her, "Jyoti, you just came here. Jet lag is affecting your mood. Let's stay here for a while, and then if you're still not happy, I promise you, we will go back." That 'for a while' sure lasted more than few days…

The doorbell rang and brought her back to the present. She lived alone now in a condo; a lot of water has passed under the bridge since their days in Decatur. Her neighbors were waiting for her to join them on their daily morning walk. They noticed that she was unusually quiet and asked her why, but she just smiled, lost in old memories.

She had a sudden urge to do something to honor this special day so after the walk she casually invited everybody in for tea. After walking three miles, it was very tempting for their tired legs, so everybody happily accepted. She hurriedly raided the refrigerator and found burphi and freshly cut pineapple and grabbed the banana bread from the freezer. As they settled down to sip Indian Masala chai, she casually asked everybody,

"So, do you remember where you were and what you were doing exactly 50 years ago today? I do."

***

Postscript - August 2017

After waiting almost three years since Madhukar's death, I received a letter from the Framingham Heart study with the lab results from Madhukar's brain donation. The results told me Madhukar did not have Alzheimer's but Corticobasal Degeneration, or 'CBD'. I was shocked hearing that. I was puzzled because all through his sickness, he had been diagnosed with Alzheimer's disease. Corticobasal degeneration was very rare, with less than five people per 100,000 and also had no cure. I remember Dr. Nair always told me that nobody is sure of Alzheimer's until a brain biopsy is performed. I was relieved to know CBD is not hereditary. A big heavy sword that was hanging by a hair was removed; my darling daughters would not be affected by their father's illness. The neurologist at the Framingham Heart Study assured me confidently that it doesn't matter if my memoirs referred to Madhukar's illness throughout as Alzheimer's Disease, because CBD's symptoms are extremely similar to Alzheimer's.

Acknowledgements

It has taken a village to write this book. I have been so fortunate for all the people I met on my journey and will be forever grateful to them. Not everyone can be named here, for that would fill another book, but I must mention a few: My two elder brothers - Prabhakar Deodhar, who gave me his listening ears, and Dilip Deodhar, who became my lighthouse, giving my writing direction. I was also fortunate to have the constant encouragement of the late Mr. Gumaste, my schoolteacher, whom I reconnected with after more than 50 years. Last but not least, my darling daughters, Swati and Chitra, who urged me to translate my original book from Marathi into English. They helped me with the immense and very emotional task of editing this book.

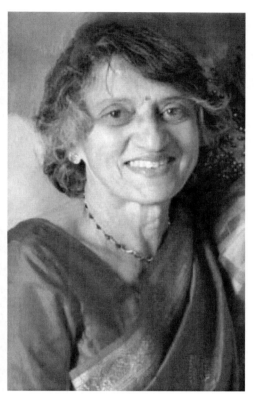

Jyoti Joshi was born in Mumbai and came to the United States as a newlywed 54 years ago. She received her Bachelor of Arts from Sir J.J. School of Art in Mumbai, has held solo exhibitions, and has won numerous awards in juried competitions. Jyoti was a preschool teacher for 23 years, during which time she also conducted workshops for parents and teachers. She has been teaching yoga and stress management classes since 1982. Jyoti's short stories, poems, and articles, written in her native language of Marathi, have been published in India and North America. Her previous book, Patazad, is inspired by correspondence with her mother. This book, The Journey of Seven Steps, was initially published in Marathi. Jyoti resides in Massachusetts near her daughters and family.

Made in United States
North Haven, CT
25 October 2021